INTELLECTUAL DISABILITIES

Other titles in the
Systemic Thinking and Practice Series
edited by David Campbell & Ros Draper
published and distributed by Karnac

Asen, E., Neil Dawson, N., & McHugh, B. *Multiple Family Therapy: The Marlborough Model and Its Wider Applications*
Bentovim, A. *Trauma-Organized Systems. Systemic Understanding of Family Violence: Physical and Sexual Abuse*
Boscolo, L., & Bertrando, P. *Systemic Therapy with Individuals*
Burck, C., & Daniel, G. *Gender and Family Therapy*
Campbell, D., Draper, R., & Huffington, C. *Second Thoughts on the Theory and Practice of the Milan Approach to Family Therapy*
Campbell, D., Draper, R., & Huffington, C. *Teaching Systemic Thinking*
Campbell, D., & Grønbæk, M. *Taking Positions in the Organization*
Campbell, D., & Mason, B. (Eds.) *Perspectives on Supervision*
Cecchin, G., Lane, G., & Ray, W. A. *The Cybernetics of Prejudices in the Practice of Psychotherapy*
Cecchin, G., Lane, G., & Ray, W. A. *Irreverence: A Strategy for Therapists' Survival*
Dallos, R. *Interacting Stories: Narratives, Family Beliefs, and Therapy*
Draper, R., Gower, M., & Huffington, C. *Teaching Family Therapy*
Farmer, C. *Psychodrama and Systemic Therapy*
Flaskas, C., Mason, B., & Perlesz, A. *The Space Between: Experience, Context, and Process in the Therapeutic Relationship*
Flaskas, C., & Perlesz, A. (Eds.) *The Therapeutic Relationship in Systemic Therapy*
Fredman, G. *Death Talk: Conversations with Children and Families*
Hildebrand, J. *Bridging the Gap: A Training Module in Personal and Professional Development*
Hoffman, L. *Exchanging Voices: A Collaborative Approach to Family Therapy*
Jones, E. *Working with Adult Survivors of Child Sexual Abuse*
Jones, E., & Asen, E. *Systemic Couple Therapy and Depression*
Krause, I.-B. *Culture and System in Family Therapy*
Mason, B., & Sawyerr, A. (Eds.) *Exploring the Unsaid: Creativity, Risks, and Dilemmas in Working Cross-Culturally*
Robinson, M. *Divorce as Family Transition: When Private Sorrow Becomes a Public Matter*
Seikkula, J., & Arnkil, T. E. *Dialogical Meetings in Social Networks*
Smith, G. *Systemic Approaches to Training in Child Protection*
Wilson, J. *Child-Focused Practice: A Collaborative Systemic Approach*

Work with Organizations

Campbell, D. *Learning Consultation: A Systemic Framework*
Campbell, D. *The Socially Constructed Organization*
Campbell, D., Coldicott, T., & Kinsella, K. *Systemic Work with Organizations: A New Model for Managers and Change Agents*
Campbell, D., Draper, R., & Huffington, C. *A Systemic Approach to Consultation*
Cooklin, A. *Changing Organizations: Clinicians as Agents of Change*
Haslebo, G., & Nielsen, K. S. *Systems and Meaning: Consulting in Organizations*
Huffington, C., & Brunning, H. (Eds.) *Internal Consultancy in the Public Sector: Case Studies*
McCaughan, N., & Palmer, B. *Systems Thinking for Harassed Managers*
Oliver, C. *Reflexive Inquiry: A Framework for Consultancy Practice*

Credit Card orders, Tel: +44 (0) 20-8969-4454; Fax: +44 (0) 20-8969-5585
Email: shop@karnacbooks.com

INTELLECTUAL DISABILITIES
A Systemic Approach

Edited by
Sandra Baum and Henrik Lynggaard

Foreword by
Tom Andersen

Systemic Thinking and Practice Series

Series Editors
David Campbell & Ros Draper

KARNAC

First published in 2006 by
H. Karnac Books Ltd.
118 Finchley Road, London NW3 5HT

Copyright © 2006 by Sandra Baum and Henrik Lynggaard
Foreword Copyright © 2006 by Tom Andersen

The rights of the editors and contributors to be identified as the authors of this work have been asserted in accordance with §§ 77 and 78 of the Copyright Design and Patents Act 1988.

All rights reserved. No part of this publication may be reproduced, stored in a retrieval system, or transmitted, in any form or by any means, electronic, mechanical, photocopying, recording, or otherwise, without the prior written permission of the publisher.

British Library Cataloguing in Publication Data

A C.I.P. for this book is available from the British Library

ISBN-13: 978-1-85575-316-7
ISBN-10: 1-85575-316-2

Edited, designed, and produced by Communication Crafts

www.karnacbooks.com

CONTENTS

SERIES EDITORS' FOREWORD   vii

ACKNOWLEDGEMENTS   ix

ABOUT THE EDITORS AND CONTRIBUTORS   xi

FOREWORD
    Tom Andersen   xv

INTRODUCTION   xix

1   Working systemically with intellectual disability: why not?
    Glenda Fredman   1

2   The use of the systemic approach to adults with intellectual disabilities and their families: historical overview and current research
    Sandra Baum   21

3   Lifespan family therapy services
    Sabrina Halliday and Lorna Robbins   42

4	Setting up and evaluating a family therapy service in a community team for people with intellectual disabilities *Sandra Baum and Sarah Walden*	64
5	Engaging people with intellectual disabilities in systemic therapy *Denise Cardone and Amanda Hilton*	83
6	New stories of intellectual disabilities: a narrative approach *Katrina Scior and Henrik Lynggaard*	100
7	Supporting transitions *Jennifer Clegg and Susan King*	120
8	Who needs to change? Using systemic ideas when working in group homes *Selma Rikberg Smyly*	142
9	The practitioner's position in relation to systemic work in intellectual disability contexts *Helen Pote*	164
10	So how do I . . . ? *Henrik Lynggaard and Sandra Baum*	185

| *REFERENCES* | 203 |
| *INDEX* | 221 |

SERIES EDITORS' FOREWORD

This book opens a door to a client group that has not, until now, had the benefit of the application of systemic thinking to its dilemmas and challenges. It is timely on this occasion to pause and consider why so little has been written in this area. The contributors to this book would probably agree that services for this client group are often under-resourced or overlooked. It is not a group that speaks vociferously for its own rights; it is called by some the "Cinderella service" in the mental health field. Intellectual disability, also referred to as learning disability, has traditionally been thought of as primarily a cognitive process rather than a complex process of fitting a particular individual into the environment around him or her.

But here, the editors, Sandra Baum and Henrik Lynggaard, have assembled the work of colleagues who have been quietly working with intellectually disabled clients, their families, and the institutions that provide their care. We say "quietly" because Baum and Lynggaard recognized that practitioners were doing sophisticated work in isolation from each other and that the time had come to present a body of theory and practice to the mental health field. We find these contributions fresh and full of enthusiasm for the work.

The ten chapters cover topics that range from a thorough, scholarly review of the specific systemic ideas applied in the book; to the principles for working therapeutically with this client group; to working with narrative models; to setting up a family therapy service in the community; and to the use of systemic ideas when consulting to group homes. Reading the book gives one both a richer sense of the issues that practitioners face in this difficult work and also a fuller appreciation of the flexible application of systemic thinking, not only to the client group but to the various ways therapists can understand and then position themselves within society's complicated value system about care for the intellectually disabled.

Readers of this Series will know that systemic practitioners are also saying more about the self-reflexivity they bring to their therapeutic relationships, and these authors have stopped to reflect on what it means for them personally to be working with this client group and how this understanding may affect the way they relate to their clients, the other family members, and the professionals in the caring system.

David Campbell
Ros Draper
London, April 2006

ACKNOWLEDGEMENTS

We are indebted to David Campbell, Glenda Fredman, and Tom Andersen for their encouragement, enthusiasm, and ongoing faith in us throughout the writing of this book. We would like to thank them all for their helpful comments and guidance, which have been much appreciated.

We would like to thank all the contributors to this book for their patience with us over many months as the book was shaped and re-shaped.

We are grateful to Jo Bownas for her helpful suggestions on several sections of the book. Thanks to Kathy Chaney, Head Librarian at Salomons Canterbury Christchurch University College, for help with the references. We also appreciate the BPS, DCP Faculty for Learning Disabilities for supporting us to organize two national conferences. These allowed us to exchange and develop ideas on working systemically. We would also like to acknowledge our respective employers, Newham Primary Care Trust and Camden & Islington Mental Health and Social Care Trust, in continuing to support our ongoing professional development, of which the editing of this book is one aspect.

Most of all, we extend our thanks to all of our clients who have contributed to our learning through generously sharing their stories and experiences with all of us. Throughout this book when we have used examples from our practice, we have used pseudonyms to protect their privacy.

Last, but by no means least, on a personal note we would like to thank our respective partners, Nick Tiratsoo and Simon Fieldman, for understanding that time had to be carved out of numerous weekends in order to make the completion of this book possible.

Sandra Baum and Henrik Lynggaard

ABOUT THE EDITORS AND CONTRIBUTORS

Sandra Baum is a Consultant Clinical Psychologist with Newham Primary Care NHS Trust. She has a postgraduate certificate in systems approaches to families and organizations from the Tavistock Centre. Her clinical work and research interests focus on using systemic approaches with families and staff teams and on improving services for parents with intellectual disabilities.

Denise Cardone is a Consultant Clinical Psychologist with Worcestershire Mental Health Partnership NHS Trust. She has completed the intermediate level family therapy training at the Family Institute, University of Glamorgan, and systemic management training at the Tavistock Clinic. She has been running Trust-wide systemic services for men and women with intellectual disabilities since 1999. Areas of interest and research include interviewing people with intellectual disabilities, interrogative suggestibility, and person-centred approaches to therapy.

Jennifer Clegg is a Senior Lecturer at the University of Nottingham, an Honorary Consultant Clinical Psychologist with Nottinghamshire Healthcare NHS Trust, and a UKCP-registered Systemic Psychotherapist (2000–2004). Her past and current research explores the transition to adult services; she also writes about ethical and conceptual issues relevant to intellectual disabilities.

Glenda Fredman is a Consultant Clinical Psychologist in Systemic Psychotherapy with Camden and Islington Mental Health and Social Care NHS Trust and a UKCP-registered Systemic Psychotherapist. She works systemically with a range of services working with children, adults, older people, physical health, and people identified with intellectual disabilities. She is extensively involved in systemic training and supervision and is the author of *Death Talk: Conversations with Children and Families* and *Transforming Emotion: Conversations in Counselling and Psychotherapy*.

Sabrina Halliday is a Consultant Clinical Psychologist with Somerset Partnership and Social Care NHS Trust. She originally became involved in family therapy when working in child and adolescent services and then became interested in how it could be combined with other systemic processes when working with children and adults with intellectual disabilities.

Amanda Hilton is a Consultant Clinical Psychologist with Gloucestershire Partnership Trust, working with children and adults with intellectual disabilities. She organizes a county-wide service working systemically with people with intellectual disabilities, their families, and staff groups.

Susan King is a Consultant Clinical Psychologist with Nottinghamshire Healthcare NHS Trust and a UKCP-registered Systemic Psychotherapist. She was brought up in Belgium and is the third generation in her family to migrate to a different country, which gives her an interest in the many ways we negotiate between different taken-for-granted cultural realities.

Henrik Lynggaard is a Chartered Clinical Psychologist with Camden and Islington Mental Health NHS Trust in London and is currently completing his systemic psychotherapy training at KCC. He was born and brought up in Denmark but has trained and worked mainly in the UK, where he has developed a strong interest in adapting systemic and narrative approaches in his conversations with people with intellectual disabilities.

Helen Pote is a Lecturer on the Clinical Psychology Doctorate at Royal Holloway, University of London, and a Clinical Psychologist with Harrow Primary Care NHS Trust. She works clinically with children and adults with intellectual disabilities. Her research interests focus on the process and effectiveness of systemic therapies, particularly for people with intellectual disabilities.

Selma Rikberg Smyly is a Consultant Clinical Psychologist with Oxfordshire Learning Disability NHS Trust. Born and brought up in Helsinki, Finland, she trained and worked mainly in the UK but worked also for five years in Zimbabwe. She feels that her cross-cultural experiences have helped her to understand better the many and varied experiences of being part of a subculture, such as intellectual disability, and what being different can mean. Current interests include exploring systemic supervision models.

Lorna Robbins is a Chartered Clinical Psychologist with Leeds Mental Health and Teaching NHS Trust. She is in the process of completing her training to be a Systemic Psychotherapist at Leeds Family Therapy Research Centre. Her previous research explored the influence of family system factors associated with outcome in post-traumatic brain injury. Her current interests include using social constructionist and narrative approaches with staff teams and in supervision.

Katrina Scior is a Lecturer on the Clinical Psychology Doctorate at University College London and Clinical Psychologist with Newham Primary Care NHS Trust. Her clinical work and research interests focus on adolescents with intellectual disabilities and their families and on mental health problems experienced by people with intellectual disabilities.

Sarah Walden is a Chartered Clinical Psychologist with Berkshire Healthcare NHS Trust, working with children and adults with intellectual disabilities. Her research interests include parents' experiences of caring for their adult offspring with intellectual disabilities. She has a real enthusiasm for working systemically and hopes to further her systemic training with the Tavistock Clinic in the near future.

FOREWORD

Significant new voices

Tom Andersen

This book feels like a big step towards solidarity. It is freeing that the book carefully turns our usual descriptions of "them" to describing and including "us". Yes, this is a book of inclusion, and it holds the ambition that all those who have not had speaking voices, and therefore not been heard, now shall be given that possibility.

* * *

It is actually exciting to notice that the authors of this book, who have received the voices of people with intellectual disabilities, think that the words that they have heard contain something significant about the person's personal and particular meanings. Many of the "disabled peoples'" words may even embrace untold life experiences: sometimes happy, sometimes sad and painful. In one chapter we learn that those who assisted Pete let him have the silences and pauses he needed to think about what he had just said or perhaps what he might choose to say or not to say next. He spoke in short uncomplicated sentences and used words that may have multiple meanings. There are many possibilities for understanding his use of the words "cock-up" and "condition". The lead therapist resisted the temptation to find meaning according to her own ideas and biases; instead, she waited for Pete to give his own meanings in his own time. This is no less than beautiful, and on behalf of the readers I feel very thankful for this book.

* * *

Being a stranger to using the English language on a daily basis, I have found it interesting to look in my rather good English–Norwegian dictionary to find the Norwegian equivalent for a given English word. Often an English word translates into many Norwegian words. I then reverse this process to find the English words for the various Norwegian words that I come across. Since "disability" and "disabilities" appear so often in this book, I was determined to investigate these words. Moving from English to Norwegian and back again to English, I encountered the following terms: hindrance; impediment; obstacle; incompetence; uselessness; weakness; ineptitude; ineptness; disqualification. In the traditional view of a person, one thinks that what a person says and does comes from inside the person. According to this view, the "source" of hindrance; impediment; obstacle; incompetence; uselessness; weakness; ineptitude; ineptness; disqualification is somewhere inside the person. If, however, one adopts another view of what a person is—namely, that what one says and what one does are answers to what others said and did to the person—then this exchange of expressions and answers shapes who the person becomes. Therefore we can ask: with whom does the person become incompetent or weak? And we can ask: with whom does the person become competent and strong? What does that other person do? This book has answers to this, and that is what makes this book so important.

* * *

As a small gift of thanks for this book, I will mention what is done in the services for various people with disabilities in Uppsala County in Sweden. These people, their families, and the professional network meet with an "outsider" who first asks the professionals to describe their collaboration with the disabled people and their families. The disabled people and their families are then asked for their views and to comment on the collaboration with the professionals. These interviews are observed from a different room by another group of people who listen to and watch the conversation on a TV screen. This group is made up of senior representatives from different services, such as social services, education, employment, and so forth. Those who participated in the interviews are then asked to join the people in the viewing suite to hear what the service managers were thinking when they heard the conversation. Much interesting discussion occurs. The service managers do not only comment, but also ask the disabled people and their families for advice about their own professional dilemmas. Suddenly the disabled people become "supervisors" to the authorities.

* * *

When this book has sold out and is to be re-published, it would be nice if the different authors could add a section to their chapters in which they describe what happened next: the conversations they had with their clients, their families, other professionals, and managers; and how their work has progressed as a consequence.

INTRODUCTION

Who are we in this work?
Connections and reflections of the contributors

Many of us are aware that people identified with intellectual disabilities have lived marginalized and devalued lives because of the prejudiced and disabling stories told of them. It has also often been implied that, professionally, the field of intellectual disabilities constitutes a bit of a backwater. Sometimes it seems to be assumed that anyone can work in the area of intellectual disabilities, that qualifications and experience are not necessarily a requirement. Qualified practitioners who do choose to enter this area of work may, in turn, be perceived by their peers as less bright and less successful. These more or less explicitly stated assumptions are, of course, a rebounding echo of the marginalizing and devaluing discourses that surround and shape the lives of the people we work with. Given some of these erroneous, but nevertheless prevalent, assumptions, we asked ourselves in writing this book: what draws us into this work, what sustains us, and how does working in this area affect us? Many different stories, originating in the many different contexts of our lives, could undoubtedly be told in answer to these questions. In what follows we share accounts given by many of the contributors.

Some of our accounts refer to our own experiences of being in families:

> "Growing up with a cousin with autism and a good friend with Down's syndrome, I remember being curious about the different ways of us understanding and interacting with the world, long before I understood that some of these differences related to something called 'disability'."

> "I grew up with a sister with physical disabilities, and this has enabled me to experience first-hand the discrimination she has faced as well as her perseverance to live an ordinary life in spite of a lot of prejudice from other people."

> "Growing up as a hearing child of deaf parents made me very aware of the power imbalance associated with disability, how 'invisible' disabled people can be to the non-disabled population. Those experiences, as well as voluntary work with people with physical and intellectual disabilities, fuelled a strong sense of social justice in me, a need to be part of something that attempts to redress this power imbalance, that maximizes opportunities for people with intellectual disabilities to be seen and heard."

Some of us have recalled memories of working in institutions:

> "I remember starting working in a 250-bed institution in 1984 where people with learning disabilities lived in barren, impoverished, overcrowded environments. It was so rewarding to be part of the community-resettlement process, to enable these people to move out into small group homes, and for them to have their own bedrooms for the first time at 50 years of age!"

> "I started work in 1975 in a 2,000-bed Scottish hospital and know that the vast majority of people managed in such environments now have lives that are changed out of all recognition."

> "I spent time with adults from the local long-stay hospital, going out with them on excursions into the community. I recall feeling humbled by seeing things that I took for granted (e.g., trips to the pub or the shops) from the perspective of someone to whom these trips were an exciting adventure or nerve-wracking journey into the unknown. Returning with people to the hospital, I recall the sense of shock and outrage at the circumstances of

their lives and realizing how much more privileged my own life was by comparison."

Some of us describe our initial apprehension
about working with this client group:

"I remember arriving at a forbidding-looking institution on a cold and rainy day for the first day of my six-month placement in learning disabilities. As I tried to find my way around the sprawling buildings, I could occasionally hear shouting and wailing coming from the inside. I recall thinking to myself, 'Thank goodness I only have to work in this area for six months.' That was 12 years ago."

"I never intended to work with people with intellectual disabilities. I started work in this area in 1995, with all the concerns and apprehensions that I see in trainees new to the field now. I did not know if I would be able to communicate with the clients. I was concerned that the work would not be interesting."

Other of our stories speak of being motivated
by a sense of social injustice:

"I was motivated by the importance of inclusion. There was my 'ordinary' youth group and the youth group for people with learning disabilities. At the ordinary group, we met in the evening, broke all the rules, and generally went unsupervised. The youth group for people with learning disabilities met on a Saturday morning (when no self-respecting teenager would even be awake), had many adults and parents attending, and had no room for teenage experimentation. It seemed odd to me then. This sense of why things are often different for people with learning disabilities, without question or choice, has stayed with me."

"Writings from the narrative-therapy field have made me consider the problems or stories that clients come to therapy with through a political lens and helped me make sense of difficulties in the context of oppressive cultural assumptions and social practices. More and more I find myself working with or seeking advice from self-advocacy groups that not only help to give people with intellectual disabilities a voice, but also work towards attitude change in the wider community."

> "What attracted me to working in this area and has kept me 'hooked' is the sense that not only do I need to draw on a wide range of psychological theories and skills, but my work is never divorced from the social context of clients' lives and the services within which we operate. It is, more than anything, the ever-present link between the personal and the political that satisfies my desire not only to make a positive change to individuals' lives, but also to tackle social injustice through clinical work and research."

> "The principles of normalization and the social model of disability politicized my understanding of disability and handicap. It was also personal, as I was invited into the lives of these young people and their families and their care staff at a time of tremendous change and commitment to a different future despite fears and risks. I met people who became unrecognizable in terms of their independence. They enjoyed going to the pub and doing their weekly shop, and they matured with the responsibility of such a life. I was struck by how much it showed in their faces as well as in their mood and behaviour. . . . The creativity and persistence of the support provided by the care staff demonstrated what could be achieved. Care staff and service users alike began to get to know each other much more as rounded individuals."

Some of us have also reflected on the question of what sustains us in this work:

> "I am sustained by the diversity of the work: in one day I can be working with an individual with intellectual disabilities, with family members, or with a team of care staff or I can be designing a service system or be negotiating between team members."

> "What sustains me in this work is very much the people that I work with. The clients themselves forever keep me on my toes, and this resonates with my early experiences of curiosity. My work life is never boring and continually challenges my perception of the world and pushes me to explore the 'taken for granted'."

> "For me this area of work is intellectually stimulating. It calls on so many abilities and requires us to be creative, resourceful, and flexible."

> "It is also an intellectual stretch to find ways of translating abstract ideas into concrete, understandable, useable forms, for clients, for their families, and for the staff groups who work with them."

> "I know a man who is blind and fractures his bones easily if he starts thrashing about in anger—he can scream and self-injure for three hours at a time. Yet when he is accompanied by familiar and thoughtful people and engaged with them on things he enjoys, his joyful comments and remarkable ability to mimic voices really enliven social events. I enjoy working with others to create the patterns of support that maintain such transformations."

> "What makes the work exciting and interesting is that it constantly requires me to be learning new things, to apply the knowledge that I have of developmental psychology and psychological therapy, and to understand change at the micro-level as well as the macro-level, to always remain open-minded, and not to presume to know but to be curious and to really find out about people's experiences and perspectives."

Other accounts describe our relationship to abilities and disabilities:

> "Working with people who have life-long disabilities can be painful and sad. It evokes feelings such as 'are we doing enough?'"

> "At times the use of language and metaphor by the people I have worked with has been poetic. At other times it has been the silence of their trauma that has spoken to me and tested my ability 'to be with' their pain and loss."

> "One day I was sitting in a session with a client. Between us, on a low table, we had spread out a large sheet of paper on which I was noting some of the skills he was telling me had helped him overcome difficulties in his life. Suddenly he said: 'Don't you write quickly? I wish I could do that!' I stopped in my tracks and made some clumsy inconsequential remark. But at that point my attention was suddenly drawn to one of the differences in abilities between us. In my work there are times when I am suddenly aware of the socially valued ways in which I am more able than many of the people I work with. However, there are other times when I am acutely aware of my inability to connect with or communicate with people. This area of work has certainly made me aware of the waxing and waning of abilities, and how these are informed and shaped by many different contexts and situations."

"As my journey working with people with intellectual disabilities has developed over time, so have my personal circumstances. Key transition points in my own life, such as getting married and having children, have been the times when I've been most acutely aware of some of the differences between myself and some of the people with intellectual disabilities and their carers I've worked with. These are the times when I've had the most complicated and difficult feelings about working in this area."

"Society values certain abilities very highly. The term 'intellectual disabilities' seems restrictive and narrow. It leaves out so many aspects of what makes a life—'emotional intelligence', to mention just one thing. I have met many people with so-called intellectual disabilities who have grasped the emotional temperature of a situation much more quickly than other so-called non-disabled people. For example, I remember a young woman with a significant degree of learning disabilities who, on several occasions, got tissues out from her pocket well before either my co-worker or I had any idea that her mother was about to cry."

"By its very nature, being a therapist usually means meeting with people who are struggling with some sort of issue or difficulty at this point in their lives. Sometimes it is easy to forget about the fun times had, for example, at theme parks, swimming, bowling, discos, etc. when working as a support worker. Recently someone whom I had been working with attended the session with her boyfriend. The playful banter between them, shared love of Elvis, and stories about a recent holiday and events at work presented a much richer and more colourful picture of her life. I couldn't remember a time when my office had been filled with so much laughter. So, added to her survivor's story, were now vibrant stories of her as a rock-and-roll fan, friend, and partner."

"It is difficult to describe the positives of working with people who have intellectual disability without romanticizing them and their lives. People with intellectual disability do not have special access to truth. They do challenge us to meet them where they are and give us a profound sense of encounter when we manage to do so. Such intense encounters help us to know ourselves and the world differently."

"One of the themes that has come up on a number of occasions in my work with people with intellectual disabilities has been their sense of 'them and us'. One young man described feelings of anger and depression connected to realizations that life-events that those around him took for granted (e.g., *marriage, children, learning to drive) were unlikely to be a part of his experience. Part of our work together was to try to find ways for him to talk to other people about his feelings, and in a manner that could be heard and acknowledged. His insightful comments, whilst painful and challenging, have encouraged me to talk much more with people about their experience of disability and the impact of this on their sense of identity, masculinity, and femininity."*

Why have we used the term "intellectual disabilities"?

For the purposes of this book we have elected to use the term "intellectual disabilities" to refer to people who come into contact with our services. All the contributors work in the UK, where the terms "learning disabilities" or "learning difficulties" are in common use, but we realize that these terms have rather different meanings beyond our own shores. We also realize that, in our own context, the term "learning disabilities" is not without its problems and that most of the service users we come into contact with prefer to be identified, first and foremost, as "people".

The International Association for the Scientific Study of Intellectual Disabilities (IASSID), an interdisciplinary scientific nongovernmental organization with official relations with the World Health Organization, has promoted the term "intellectual disabilities" in an attempt to foster consistency and dialogue across different countries. IASSID promotes worldwide research and exchange of information on intellectual disabilities. However, as with all previous terms used to make distinctions between groups of people, "intellectual disabilities" is not without its problems. In many Western societies intellect is held in high regard. The *Concise Oxford Dictionary* defines intellectual as "possessing a high level of understanding or intelligence; cultured" and intellect as "the faculty of reasoning, knowing, and thinking, as distinct from feeling." The faculties associated with "intellect" therefore seem to have more to do with inherent properties of the skin-bounded self, whereas a concept of "learning" seems to encompass a notion of social activity and social relatedness. As is pointed out by both Glenda Fredman and Sandra Baum in chapters one and two, respectively, the terms "intellectual" or "learning" are bound up with cultural norms and contexts, valuing particular aspects of what it means to be a person while devaluing others. Similarly, the term "disabilities" is problematic if it is considered as a property solely residing within the person without reference to the interrelation between the person and societal responses that magnify, or in some situations create, the disability.

In the light of these considerations it has been a struggle for us to decide how to refer to the people who use our services. From a professional perspective we wanted to communicate with people across the world, but from a personal perspective we are mindful of the moral and relational consequences of using the different labels (in terms of how people get positioned, how they are identified, how they come to see themselves, and how they are valued and treated). Many of the contributors to this book have reservations about using the term "intellectual disabilities", as it is rarely used in day-to-day interaction with the people with whom we work or with our colleagues in this country. Nevertheless, we recognize the need to join all those languages that allow us to be in dialogue with others. Therefore, in order to include colleagues across the world in this conversation we are—here and for now—electing to use this terminology.

The intentions of the book

In writing this book it has been our intention to bring together the contributions of a group of practitioners from all over the UK who have been using systemic approaches in their work. We hope it will inspire others to try out different ways of working and being with people with intellectual disabilities and their wider systems. We also hope that systemic practitioners who are unfamiliar with this client group might give consideration to extending their practice to also work with people with intellectual disabilities. Two of our contributors have commented that:

> "Having lived and worked with people with intellectual disabilities all of my life, when I came to study psychology, I found that the theories and models (behavioural, cognitive) didn't ring true; although there may have been some useful ideas, I felt that they did not reflect my lived experience. They ignored relationship (in the broadest and most important sense of the word). When I looked at the literature on fami-

lies and people with intellectual disabilities, I found it pejorative—only about problems like high stress levels, the toll it took on marriages, siblings in distress, etc. I found second-order family therapy ideas much more affirming, and I think they show a more ethical way of working."

"Therapeutically, I think systemic family therapy's long-term engagement with difference, rather than with erasing difference, will make an important contribution to the creation of fruitful dialogue that allows my intellectual life and my clients' intellectual lives to engage with one another. . . . Qualifying as a systemic family therapist and then interpreting those ideas for the particular needs encountered in intellectual disability services has been a significant intellectual task."

We hope that you, too, may find something in this book that "rings true"; that is affirming and inspiring; that invites you to a rewarding engagement with difference; and that is "intellectually significant".

CHAPTER ONE

Working systemically with intellectual disability: why not?

Glenda Fredman

*I*t is the start of the 1970s. I am an undergraduate student spending a few days at an institution accommodating people called "mentally retarded". To occupy me, the institution staff have suggested I take David off for the day and teach him to tie his shoelaces. David's slipper-type footwear does not have laces. He tells me these are his only shoes. Intent on performing the task set for me, I find us some string and prepare to teach David to tie a bow!

First I identify appropriate rewards for David. I learn from David that he likes to eat apples and cheese. Guided by the principles of behaviourism, I proceed to break down "bow-tying" into small steps or sub-skills. Then, rewarding David with small pieces of apple and cheese for successive approximations of the sub-skills of bow tying, through shaping and chaining, I "train" him to tie a bow. David seems very content to pass the day with me in this manner. The institution staff, on the other hand, appear unsettled that we are still in each other's company when I escort David to lunch and then collect him again an hour and a half later. They seem stunned when, at the end of the day, David and I seek out their audience to demonstrate his bow-tying. I get a grade A from the university for my paper entitled "Training a Mentally Retarded Man Using Behavioural Methods".

* * *

In the second chapter of this book, Sandra Baum tracks over time the language and terminology used to describe people with intellectual disabilities. She also relates the changing definitions of intellectual disability over time to developments in service provision and philosophies of care for these so-described people. When I worked with David he was called "mentally retarded", and along with this description of his identity came a set of expectations of what he was capable of doing and not doing, where he could or should live, and what he was entitled to.

This was the 1970s, when descriptions or diagnoses of "idiot", "imbecile", "feebleminded", and "moral defective" were still in the hospital records of people like David, and the focus was more on deficiency than ability or possibility. Behaviourism was considered the treatment of choice for people labelled "mentally retarded" at that time, and relationships between so-called retarded people and their carers went unnoticed. Hence neither my tutors nor I addressed my relationship with David or the context in which he lived. Nobody considered as unethical my submitting David to learning a meaningless, useless activity; performing in front of bored staff; or objectifying him for the purposes of a psychology undergraduate's learning experience. Neither did anybody notice that David seemed to enjoy my company and attention, that he was able to spend several hours engaging with me despite his "poor attention span", nor that he had learnt a complex, albeit useless, task that was considered way beyond his intellectual capability. That David and I had enjoyed many warm giggles and handshakes (accompanied at first with bits of cheese and apple!) only minimally assuages some of the immense discomfort I still hold for engaging this young man in a pointless activity with no clear useful purpose to himself.

* * *

Moving forward to the early 1980s, I am now a trainee clinical psychologist working for six months in a large hospital for people identified as "mentally handicapped". These people are not sick but live in a hospital. They are no longer "mentally retarded", we are told, but "mentally handicapped". Again, with this description come rights, obligations, and duties for these "patients"—as they are often still called—and their carers. As a trainee clinical psychologist at this time, it is compulsory to "do" a six-month placement "in Mental Handicap". For the majority of trainees in my year, this is the least favoured placement. Most of us have booked as much leave as we are entitled to take during this placement so that we can complete just the required seventy-two days. What we dread—and many of us approach this placement with "dread"—is the institution, not the people. My supervisor has given me a book in which Frank Thomas writes about his experience as a nurse from inside an institution for mentally handicapped people (Ryan & Thomas, 1980). His account is chilling to read—the more so since it is still happening in the early 1980s. The power of Frank's story deeply touches me and moves me. His story resonates with the experiences I am having at the hospital. It reassures me that I am not going mad—no one else seems to see, hear, and feel what I do. But the book also saddens me. Despite Frank Thomas having had his account published, things remain the same.

Each day I trudge up the hill to the "back wards", as they are called, in the grounds of the hospital, set in the beautiful Hertfordshire countryside. Often it is snowing. I am clad in a thick second-hand trench coat, and my feet are freezing. Supervisors never work in the "back wards" themselves—that is where they send trainees. I pass middle-aged women pushing dolls' prams and talking to themselves. I guess they got there as "moral defectives" in their day. Waiting to speak to a nurse in one of the locked wards, where the nurses always carry huge bunches of keys attached to their belts, like prison wardens, I witness men and women between the ages of 20 and 35 in ill-fitting clothes. They are queuing up for medication, and then returning to rock and sway in corners. There is always the stench of urine and some other indeterminable sweet–stale smell—even the water tastes funny.

I ache physically and emotionally the entire six months I work at this hospital. And that does not include the days I had to have hepatitis B injections because a "Hep. B carrier" scratched me—no one told me to take care, so I allowed far more physical contact than anyone else did. Or the day I was hit in the face by a young woman whom I naively went to console, having witnessed her tearful withdrawal and then head-banging following an episode of taunting and mocking by two young nurses.

* * *

What Sandra Baum tells us in chapter two is that changing historical, political, and social contexts continually modify how and whom we define with intellectual disabilities and the language we use to describe them. We learn from her chapter that these definitions have always been conceived of by people in power. They are never the words chosen by a group of people describing or finding their own identity. Making distinctions between other people with language is never neutral. People distinguished with "mental retardation", "mental handicap", or "intellectual disability" have mostly been seen negatively, as a problem to themselves and to others. These terms are used for extremely different presentations of ability, which is a source of pain to those described who find it difficult to differentiate themselves as individuals in the eyes of others and to escape others' stereotypes of them.

The medicalization of intellectual disability has been the main instrument for excluding people from society. The medical model has invited us to focus on the difference between these people and ourselves rather than on the similarities. The authors in this book keep us mindful of the exclusion these people endure. With "normalization" (Wolfensberger, 1972) we were encouraged towards reducing difference rather than exaggerating difference and towards inclusion rather than exclusion. The authors of this book are writing in the context of "valuing people" (the title of an English White Paper: Department of Health, 2001). They acknowledge the difference of people identified with intellectual disabilities when it offers resources, also taking care to appreciate their equality to ourselves so that we do not disqualify them from the ways of living we take as our human rights. The authors of this book have found that the systemic approach offers the possibilities of enabling and empowering the people they work with to access their rights to independence, choice, inclusion, respect, and accessibility. Sabrina Halliday and Lorna Robbins (chapter three) set up their lifespan service with social inclusion as a primary intention. They noted an absence of family therapy services for devalued groups and wanted to offer the choice of family therapy services to people with intellectual disabilities who traditionally would not have easy access to this form of therapy.

What is systemic?

Like the language used to connote "intellectual disability", the word "systemic" holds many meanings that have changed and evolved over time according to historical and political contexts. Freedman and Combs (1996) identify different metaphors across different phases of systemic developments that guide the thinking and practice of systemic practitioners, both highlighting and obscuring what they attend to. The use of the word "phase" here is intended to connote continuity rather than discontinuity. Therefore it implies that systemic principles and practices have emerged during a particular phase and then continued to evolve and influence practice in different ways over time. Hence I am not suggesting that systemic ideas or practices identified as emerging during one phase are viewed as fixed in that time or history or seen as out of use in current practice.

* * *

I was first introduced to systemic practice during what Dallos and Draper (2000) refer to as the "first phase", when systemic practice was informed by the discourses of modernism, positivism, and structuralism. During this phase, commonly referred to as "first-order cybernetics", we were using the metaphor of physical systems to guide our practice and were informed by the family systems paradigm. What most engaged me with the systemic approach at that time was the emphasis on pattern and process and hence the recognition that the whole was much more than the sum of its parts. What I particularly appreciated was the focus on relationships, communication, and interaction—that is, what was happening between people rather than within people—since this moved us away from pathologizing individuals and towards viewing symptoms as interpersonal. In our practice we were therefore moving away from organizing events into linear sequences so that they could provide us with neat cause-and-effect explanations of problems, towards identifying circular patterns that connected symptoms with relationships and communication (Watzlawick, Beavin, & Jackson, 1967).

At this time we saw systems as stable and unchanging, so that our approach to family systems was somewhat mechanical. We focused on how families became "stuck" in repetitive loops of redundant behaviour or in inappropriate hierarchical structures that were unbalanced. We designed interventions for therapists to interrupt those patterns and guide families into healthy rather than unhealthy stability. With its emphasis on a functionalist view of problems, first-order cybernetics was inviting me to treat dysfunction as the focus of therapy at this time.

Using physical systems and "structure" as guiding metaphors in this way, we approached families akin to machines and therapists as something like repairers (Hoffman, 1988) whose job it was to design appropriate interventions to change the existing family structure.

Assuming that we were quite separate from the people we worked with, we saw ourselves as therapists capable of making detached, objective assessments of what was wrong and fixing people's problems like a mechanic fixes a faulty thermostat. Thus I found the cybernetic metaphor inviting me to treat clients as objects about whom I knew the truth. This objectification in turn risked inviting clients into a relationship in which I positioned myself as the knower, as the expert, and the client as the powerless, passive recipient needing my expertise.

In the 1970s and early 1980s most adults identified or, indeed, diagnosed as mentally retarded or mentally handicapped who were receiving psychological services were living in institutions. Since first-order cybernetics focused on the family, and commonly the nuclear family, rather than the wider system, systemic theory and practice seemed to pass by practitioners working with "mental retardation" at this time. The ethos of first-order cybernetics, with its focus on dysfunction, conflicted with the highly valued ethos of "normalization" in the 1980s, so that once again systemic theory and practice did not connect with our work with people identified with "mental handicap".

* * *

The authors of this book do not fully embrace *all* the systemic approaches, methods, and techniques informed by first-order cybernetics, perhaps because of the poor fit of some of these with their preferred ethical position that emphasizes valuing people and avoiding a focus on dysfunction. Also they work beyond the nuclear family to include carers and wider networks of significant relationships, with a commitment to including and giving voice to people with intellectual disabilities. However, throughout the book we see how some of the core ideas and practices emerging in this phase continue to be used and have evolved in different ways to inform current practice. For example these authors develop and incorporate into their practice the focus on context, relationships, communication, and interaction—that is, what happens between people rather than within people—which emerged in this first phase of systemic developments to distinguish systemic practice from other linear therapeutic approaches. Below, to whet your appetite, I share some examples of how these authors have used the concepts of *context, communication, connections* (in relationship), and *circularity* from this first phase.

* * *

I completed my formal training in systemic family therapy during the second phase, which we have now come to refer to as "second-order cybernetics" (e.g., see Boscolo, Cecchin, Hoffman, & Penn, 1987; Campbell, Draper, & Huffington, 1991). Systemic practitioners at this time were acknowledging that the therapist could not stand outside the family system and gain an objective view of the situation. Instead, the therapist was seen as a part of the therapy system. Hence there was a move away from the idea that anyone could perceive an objective reality towards a valuing of multiple perspectives. With this shift we began to adopt less of an expert position with clients and to see ourselves more as co-participants in the same system as family members, intending to explore collaboratively with them rather than fix or solve their problems.

Instead of the metaphors of machines and thermostats, therefore, systemic therapists started thinking in terms of biological and ecological systems and of systems as continually changing and co-evolving rather than as fixed or stable. As therapists, therefore, we began to expect and attend to how systems were changing rather than how they were "stuck". Whereas within the family systems paradigm we expected to be able to predict the behaviour of family members, from within the ecological systems paradigm we recognized human biological systems as far more complex than machines. Thus we intended to engage clients in the exploration of hypotheses from a position of curiosity (Cecchin, 1987) so as to introduce difference and open space for change. Consequently we were less intent on reaching *our* predetermined goals and more concerned to check that we were moving in the preferred directions of our clients. Instead of focusing only on patterns of behaviour, we began also to explore patterns of meaning and became curious about how meanings were constructed. During this phase we read papers by Karl Tomm (1984a, 1984b), who encouraged us to notice the interventive effects of circular questions, which could invite people to become observers to their own systems, and to attend to the interconnectedness between people in their system.

We also worked more in teams, valuing the multiple perspectives available from colleagues intending to generate together rich repertoires of ideas that we could float lightly in therapeutic conversations via the vehicle of circular questions (Tomm, 1988) and reflecting-team conversations (Andersen, 1987). Having moved away from the assumption of an objective reality "out there" about which we could learn the truth, we acknowledged that we were constructing the world through our personal, subjective lenses. Hence we were attending more to how our personal beliefs and prejudices contributed to our work with clients (Cecchin, Lane, & Ray, 1994). In this way, self-reflexivity presented a potential resource for change in our work with clients.

Much of the practice shared by the authors of this book is guided by systemic principles generated during this second-order-cybernetics phase. Later, I shall point to examples of their valuing *multiple perspectives* and their working in *collaboration* with clients and their significant systems as *co-participants* from a posture of respectful *curiosity* rather than as experts from a posture of expert knowing.

* * *

Although the authors of this book promote the valuing of multiple perspectives, they are also aware of the risk of being seduced into the sort of relativism that can deny differences in power and opportunity afforded people disadvantaged by intellectual disabilities. In retrospect we now recognize that both first- and second-order systemic explanations were guided by normative models of family life. There was no attention to differentials of power within families, with almost an implicit assumption of equal power for everyone regardless of age, ability, gender, class, race, and culture. The authors of this book are constantly mindful of the effects of the values within institutions, society, and the wider culture on the lives and relationships of people affected by intellectual disabilities. Hence they are constantly negotiating the tension between adopting respectful postures of curiosity with people in therapeutic conversations and taking positions of advocacy for their clients against discriminating, damaging, and self-diminishing values and practices. In this way a lot of the work reflected in this book is coherent with the ethics of the third, or postmodern, phase of systemic developments informed by social constructionism. (For examples of postmodern systemic practices, see McNamee & Gergen, 1992; Cronen & Lang, 1994; Griffith & Elliot Griffith, 1994; Lang & McAdam, 1995; Freedman & Combs, 1996; Fredman, 2004.) During this phase we think in terms of a linguistic systems paradigm rather than the biological or ecological systems paradigm of second-order cybernetics, and we use the narrative metaphor to guide us. Central to this worldview is the notion that we construct our realities in conversations and relationships with others and that these realities are constituted through language and maintained through narratives. Hence there is no essential truth but only knowledges that arise within communities of knowers (Freedman & Combs, 1996). In this sense, then, "intellectual disability" is not an objective phenomenon but a construction, a label given to certain actions, which consequently constitutes the identities of some people within a culture. (This is not to say that these constructions do not have real effects.) Recognizing that people identified with intellectual disabilities have less (if any) power than others to choose and construct their identities, the authors of this book take care not to reproduce in therapy the oppression many of these people have experienced within the dominant culture. Hence they are committed to *include all voices* of people involved, especially the voice of the person identified with intellectual disability. Mindful of the *power differential* inherent in all systems, they are intent on offering *choice* to people, taking into account their preferred views, and are careful to invite narratives of *competence*, ability, and resources with people whose identities are commonly constructed from dominating discourses of incompetence and inability.

* * *

I now go on to address in more detail the key systemic principles emerging from these three phases, which I recognize as guiding the work with people identified with intellectual disabilities presented in this book. I have abstracted *context, connections (in relationships), communication*, and *circularity*, which emerged in the first phase of systemic developments; *collaborative practice and curiosity about multiple perspectives*, from the second phase; and *attention to differential power, including all voices, co-creating meanings, choice, and competence*, from the third phase.

Context

Attention to context particularly distinguishes the systemic approach. Since context gives meaning to our actions, behaviour and beliefs are always examined and understood within the contexts in which they arise. Therefore, we pay specific attention to the relationship contexts of the individual—his or her family, work, group home, day centre—and recognize that these contexts are informed by the contexts of people's culture, ethnicity, race, age, ability, sexuality, and gender. John Burnham (1992) suggests the acronym DISGRACCE to help us stay mindful of the contexts of *D*isability, *I*ntellectual ability, *S*exuality, *G*ender, *R*ace, *A*ge, *C*ulture, *C*lass, and *E*thnicity.

The authors of this book note the importance of attending to context and negotiating contexts of differential power in clients' best interests within systems. In chapter two, Sandra Baum comments on the tendency of services to take an a-contextual approach, conceiving of problems as inherent within people identified with intellectual disabilities. Selma Rikberg Smyly (chapter eight) reflects on how our attitudes and beliefs are informed by our personal, familial, cultural, and social contexts and invites us to attend to the powerlessness in the lives of these people. With the example she shares, she places the problem in the context of the agency caring for the client. Katrina Scior and Henrik Lynggaard (chapter six) note that people learn in multiple contexts, "not just in an idealized nuclear family". They pay close attention to the contexts of their clients, their own contexts, and the social, cultural, and political contexts that shape the lives of them all. Helen Pote (chapter nine) identifies four levels of context that influence therapists' views of themselves and their practice with people with intellectual disability. Many authors address the context of time in terms of the family life cycle (e.g., Sandra Baum, chapter two; Jennifer Clegg & Susan King, chapter seven) taking care to avoid imposing a normative view of family development or ignoring the diversity of choice available about forms of family life, for which the first-order-cybernetics models were criticized.

Connections in relationship

With a systemic approach we are mindful that people are connected in relationship and that what one person does has an effect on other people in the system and on relationships. The authors of this book pay careful attention to relationships with clients, with referrers, and with other significant and involved members of the system. For example, Sabrina Halliday and Lorna Robbins (chapter three) highlight the relationship themes of belonging and separation, risk and protection, and responsibility. Offering interpersonal rather than individual perspectives of problems in this way, the authors of this book move away from pathologizing individuals or families and towards "working with" their clients rather than "working on" them. They give examples of asking circular questions to explore the connections between people, thereby also drawing the attention of those involved to how they are interconnected, how each person's feelings and actions are influenced by and influence the actions and feelings of the other.

Communication

Attention to communication is central to the systemic approach. In interaction it is taken that all behaviour is communication. Therefore, we "cannot not communicate" since speaking involves not only words but also action; not only the report, content, or information of what is said, but also the command implicit in the relationship between the people communicating (Watzlawick, Beavin, & Jackson, 1967).

The authors of this book pay careful attention to communication. By adjusting the pace to meet individual needs, Sabrina Halliday and Lorna Robbins (chapter three) aim to facilitate the process of communication so that family members can listen and talk to one another and feel able to express their opinions. They show how circular questioning allows each person to listen and to comment on other people's perspectives on sensitive issues in a supportive rather than confrontational context. Sandra Baum and Sarah Walden (chapter four) also tailor their language to the client's comprehension and communication abilities. Denise Cardone and Amanda Hilton (chapter five) show how someone with severe intellectual disability and communication difficulties may be engaged in a systemic process and helped to have a voice that others can hear. Cardone and Hilton, too, attend to the pace and style of therapy, use and stay close to the client's language, and modify practices such as circular questions. Thus these authors resist the temptation to attribute meanings according to their own ideas and biases, giving time for their client to give his own meanings in his own time.

Circularity

The authors of this book take the systemic perspective that beliefs and behaviour are understood as connected in a circular relationship. Hence, with a systemic approach we are mindful that attributing a cause, blame, or label to a person is a particular linear punctuation. We therefore acknowledge our responsibility to consider the ethical consequences of any linear punctuation we make. Circularity is more about pattern, interrelationship, and interaction than about cause and effect, and systemic approaches pay specific attention to the patterns that connect and the contexts that inform.

We might say that the examples at the start of this chapter reflect the linear approach to "mental retardation" and "mental handicap" of that time. Problems were attributed to the "subnormality" or incapacities of David and to the men and women rocking and swaying in corners of the institution where I trained. There was no interest in relating their behaviour or difficulties to the way other people interacted with these people or to their living environment. In contrast, throughout this book attention is paid to the social and cultural contexts that shape people's actions and beliefs and to the interdependence of people in relationship. Each person is seen as influencing the others in ongoing recursive relationships, so that looking for a starting point or cause of problems is seen as unproductive. The authors are mindful of pathologizing, linear punctuations that locate problems within the person identified with intellectual disability. They recognize that the inequalities of power affecting these people are related to wider cultural patterns of inequality, thus leading us to consider whether many of the problems facing people identified with intellectual disability are a consequence of exclusion, discrimination, or humiliation by society. Sandra Baum (chapter two) offers the alternative punctuation that society disables people by the limited and devalued experiences it offers, and Selma Rikberg Smyly (chapter eight) asks the question, "who needs to change?"

Collaborative practice

"Collaborative" is a key word associated with systemic practice, since with this approach we collaborate with colleagues, clients, and referrers so that we are usually in conversation with large numbers of people—even if not all at once. Therefore, we commonly work in teams and look for people in the system who potentially could be a collaborative resource. The authors of this book demonstrate the value of teamwork and of engaging the collaboration of the wider system.

Sabrina Halliday and Lorna Robbins (chapter three) present a wonderful example of collaboration across multiple levels of the organization. They work with immediate and extended family, direct care staff, managers, other professionals, and other teams depending on who the person and his or her immediate system see as influential to the problem. With clients, the authors consider family therapy practice a shared process, thus confirming the ability of people with intellectual disabilities to participate fully in the process. Along with families, they involve carers and professionals where appropriate, which allows them to involve different parts of the system in addressing disability discourses. As well as collaborating with secondary services and with different professional systems, they also connect with carers and service-users groups to enhance accessibility to their service. They have found that involving different parts of the system in this collaborative work has effected change in the wider system. Through participating in open dialogue with their clients, care staff started using more positive and empowering language about their clients and were able to look beyond the "disability" labels and discourses so that they could notice the abilities and involvement of the person identified with intellectual disability.

For Denise Cardone and Amanda Hilton (chapter five), working collaboratively is central to "inclusion, empowerment, engagement, and person-centred practice", which guide policies and practice in the field of intellectual disability in the UK. They emphasize that working together in a non-judgemental way is achieved not from the position of the outside expert who privileges professional knowledge, but from an acknowledgement of the subjectivity of each and every point of view. In this way they value the multiple perspectives of all involved. Katrina Scior and Henrik Lynggaard (chapter six) demonstrate this sort of collaborative practice when they invite clients identified with intellectual disabilities to teach them, thus showing their clients how their knowledges can be used to help professionals learn about challenging their sorts of problems.

Curiosity about multiple perspectives

Many of the authors of this book use versions of reflecting teams to present and value multiple perspectives. The lead practitioner interviews the clients, who may be any combinations of individuals, couples, families, care staff, or significant professionals. The team listens to the interview while they talk. At a time agreed with those being interviewed, the team talks about what they have heard, while the lead practitioner and those who were interviewed listen. This creates an opportunity for the team to offer multiple perspectives and for the family to hear different conversations and enables more egalitarian relationships between clients and practitioners. Using the language of the clients, the team talks tentatively and respectfully about what has been said (not what is not said) and offers differences that are not too unusual (Andersen, 1987; Lax, 1995). Denise Cardone and Amanda

Hilton (chapter five) offer guidelines for using reflecting teams with people with intellectual disabilities.

Selma Rikberg Smyly (chapter eight) sees her role as to enable others to solve problems, not to solve the problem on their behalf. Therefore, she engages as many relevant people from the client's network of concern as possible in a creative collaborative exercise involving reflecting conversations whereby everyone is the expert and all their contributions are important to the process of finding a way to go on. In this way, she co-creates new stories with clients and their significant networks of family and carers, incorporating expert knowledges from all involved.

Including all voices and attention to differential power

The highest context in this book is valuing people, giving people a voice. The reflecting processes described above appear to provide people with intellectual disabilities with an empowering and novel experience of being heard. These people have frequently been grouped in a category that does not acknowledge their subjectivity. Thus they have had few opportunities to be anything other than that prescribed by the definitions of self and social roles attributed to them.

Sabrina Halliday and Lorna Robbins (chapter three) are mindful that they are working with people who rarely get heard, and the authors therefore work together at a pace set by their clients towards identifying a focus for the sessions. They report that the people identified with intellectual disabilities have commented that having what they say listened to is a new and positive experience. Selma Rikberg Smyly (chapter eight) points out that people identified with intellectual disabilities commonly have their lives storied by others. She therefore works towards changing the emphasis from predominantly professional descriptions of the clients to incorporating and privileging the views of carers, family, and most importantly clients in *co-creating* new stories and meanings. Her elegant approach offers us ways to "give everyone in the room an opportunity to speak as well as to listen", so that all voices can be respected without some views dominating the meeting.

Denise Cardone and Amanda Hilton (chapter five) also demonstrate how they create a context to share and hear voices where everyone can hear each other's views. They give people identified with intellectual disabilities more opportunities and time to voice their views in relation to the others present. The result is a slower therapeutic process. This can offer the chance for the voices of people identified with intellectual disabilities—who may not be used to having a voice, especially in the presence of their carers—to be heard in a different way and their stories to be witnessed and acknowledged. Henrik Lynggaard and Sandra Baum offer further creative ways to include the voice of the person identified with intellectual disability in their concluding chapter (chapter 10).

Choice

Working in collaboration with people as co-participants rather than expert advisers implies appreciation of people's rights to choose. Sabrina Halliday and Lorna Robbins (chapter three) demonstrate belief in families' abilities by offering choice in how they work together. Katrina Scior and Henrik Lynggaard (chapter six) always ask about the person's preferred way of living, with questions such as "is that something that suits you?" Selma Rikberg Smyly (chapter eight), among others, shows how using versions of reflecting processes can offer clients a variety of views, including the opportunity to choose which ideas suit them and the chance to add their own ideas.

Competence and resources

Coherent with the spirit of normalization and "valuing people" (Department of Health, 2001), none of the authors in this book take a problem-focused approach that emphasizes dysfunction. Like Sabrina Halliday and Lorna Robbins, they aim to facilitate the process of change by attending to people's strengths, resources, and abilities. Katrina Scior and Henrik Lynggaard reflect on how their training as clinical psychologists focused their eyes on problems, limitations, and deficits, with the risk of blinding them to clients' abilities and resources. They note that stories describing people with intellectual disabilities as weak and lacking abilities are often so powerful and prevalent that it may be difficult for these people and their significant networks to construct, live, and circulate alternative stories. "The very word 'disability', with its focus on *absence* of 'ability'", they say, "derives from powerful assumptions as to what should be privileged." They share examples of narrative practices that enable the empowerment of people marginalized by diminishing discourses. With its focus on resurrecting and discovering people's abilities and resources rather than diagnosing pathology, they show how a narrative approach can offer an antidote to the labelling, diagnosing, and stigmatizing whereby problems (including "intellectual disability"!) have been located inside the person, overshadowing or obscuring their abilities or competencies.

Why not systemic?

Although this book is about how and why we *do* work systemically with people identified with intellectual disabilities, I also want to address *why not* systemic, since, sadly, it is this conversation that we most often get invited into when proposing systemic services for people in public services. I call it the *"conversation of impossibility"* (Fredman, 2001, p. 5). These conversations of impossibility reflect the discourses presented below. Although there is no evidence base for these discourses, they shape and form our practice, our services, and even the buildings we construct, so that they are used by practitioners, referrers, and managers as arguments against the systemic approach in many instances. I shall give examples of the discourses as well as show how the practices presented in this book, if we choose, could begin to challenge these discourses and thereby offer opportunities for different sorts of practice. Helen Pote (chapter nine) also offers possible systemic responses to what she calls "clinical dilemmas" emerging in the contexts of some of these discourses.

Only for the verbally articulate

The first discourse holds that systemic therapy is only for verbal, articulate, and intelligent people, so that people who have problems communicating are not able to benefit from a systemic approach. In her chapter, Sandra Baum shows us how this discourse has been used to exclude people with intellectual disabilities from psychotherapies in general on the basis that they are considered insufficiently verbal or intelligent to benefit. There is no evidence base to substantiate this discourse, and Henrik Lynggaard and Sandra Baum's useful overview (chapter 10) of how the authors of this book include people with intellectual disabilities in family sessions offers an alternative narrative.

The whole family or nothing

I have frequently heard the claim that "the person with intellectual disability is not living with his family" or "we could never get the family to attend" as rationales against a systemic approach with individuals with intellectual disabilities presenting with relationship difficulties. Here the speaker holds the assumption that we have to see the whole family to practice systemically. He or she believes that systemic therapy equals *family* therapy and therefore the whole family must be present in the room. If people are not living with their families, this speaker assumes, we cannot do family therapy.

The whole-family-or-nothing discourse is challenged by all the authors of this book who worked systemically with the system in focus, which did not necessarily include the referred person's family. They demonstrate how they are using the approach not only with whole families in *family therapy* but also with individuals (Scior & Lynggaard, chapter six); parts of a family, for example an adult brother and sister (Halliday & Robbins chapter three); consultation to residential staff in group homes (Rikberg Smyly, chapter eight); with clients and their workers in day centres (Cardone & Hilton, chapter five); and in different conversations with different parts of the network of concern (Rikberg Smyly, chapter eight).

The family is not the problem

I have often been told that, "There is nothing wrong with the family, so they do not need family therapy." This discourse holds that family therapy is for problem families and, by implication, that healthy families need not attend therapy. Unfortunately, the family-is-not-the-problem discourse has permeated not only clinical practice but also the media, preventing potentially useful referrals for family therapy. I have frequently had family members refuse to attend sessions for fear of being blamed or criticized for the problem, and some families have reported being labelled "mad" or "bad" by professionals. Many of the approaches presented in this book offer a different narrative to the family-is-not-the-problem discourse by attending to families' strengths and abilities as possible resources to the problem.

Not for the poor or marginalized

I have frequently met the argument that systemic therapy is not suitable for inner-city, multicultural, busy public services or with poor people who are marginalized. This discourse seems to include the assumption that the systemic approach is unusual and threatening and particularly unfamiliar to people who are ethnic minorities in Britain. All the authors in this book tell a different narrative. All of the therapy examples in this book describe work with people who are marginalized, and several of the services described have been developed in poor and/or busy, multicultural inner-city areas (e.g., Baum & Walden, chapter four; Scior & Lynggaard, chapter six).

No resources (room, time, team, video)

"No room big enough" is the reason I most commonly meet for practitioners seeing no more than the single individual person when working in public services. I agree that it is not ideal to have four family members sitting perched on the GP's examining bed, or for the grandmother and therapist to sit on the floor so that the disabled family members can use the chairs, or for a practitioner with nineteen people from an extended family to "squat" in an unused hospital ward. (All of these situations actually resulted in very successful outcomes for the people who attended therapy with my colleagues and me.)

Despite evidence to the contrary, we seem to be dominated by the assumption that we have to have considerable material resources—for example, a one-way screen, team, video, and so forth—to practice systemically. The authors in this book show that it is not the equipment but, rather, the commitment of practitioners and management that makes this approach viable. They point to management support, systemic consultation, and/or supervision to their systemic service, as well as good links with the wider professional network, as key factors enabling their systemic practice.

Only qualified family therapists can do it

Many times I have witnessed the only-qualified-family-therapists-can-do-it discourse paralyse the enthusiasm and commitment of practitioners who want to introduce systemic practice into their services. The discourse implies that practitioners should practice only cognitive behavioural or psychodynamic therapies, since they are not *qualified* to do family therapy.

If we were to distinguish "working systemically" from "family therapy" and "systemic psychotherapy" in the same way that we distinguish "working psychodynamically" from "psychoanalysis" and "analytic psychotherapy", we might begin to undo the double-bind that this only-qualified-family-therapists-can-do-it discourse presents to people working with intellectual disabilities. More aptly claiming that "only qualified family therapists can work as *qualified* family therapists" might liberate practitioners to work effectively, as Sandra Baum and Sarah Walden do, in teams with families. They use supervision and/or consultation to ensure that their practice remains ethical and coherent with the systemic approach and do not lay claims to *being* family therapists.

A weak evidence base

It is the "weak-evidence-base" discourse that commonly bolsters the view that cognitive behavioural and psychodynamic therapies are the primary therapies whereas systemic therapy is experimental and unsupported by research. In their final chapter, Henrik Lynggaard and Sandra Baum offer some challenges to this weak-evidence-base discourse. As well as mentioning some qualitative studies exploring systemic work with intellectual disability, they address the need to adopt research paradigms that are commensurate with the paradigm informing systemic practice. They offer, as an example, approaching the process of therapy as co-research with clients, whereby narrative practitioners and clients have contributed accounts of their therapy together to form "archives" for the benefit of others facing similar difficulties.

In the year 2000, Sandra Baum organized a conference in London (on behalf of the British Psychological Society's Faculty for Learning Disabilities), to bring together people working systemically in the area of intellectual disabilities. One hundred people attended the conference, and many authors in this book shared moving examples of their systemic practice with people with intellectual disabilities and their families, carers, and significant networks. Services for people with intellectual disabilities had previously not been commonly associated with this approach. At this conference, presenters and participants challenged all of the above discourses of impossibility previously dogging ethical systemic work with people with intellectual disabilities in the public health services. Sandra Baum and Henrik Lynggaard have now taken another step forward. They have brought together in this book a valuable collection of creative and ethical accounts of systemic practices with people facing intellectual disability. This book therefore offers an impressive start to building "archives" of practice-based evidence of systemic approaches in the area of intellectual disabilities.

Things won't be the same

Over thirty-five years ago, Jay Haley (1975) gave mental health services several reasons for avoiding the introduction of family therapy. He warned that there would be confusion in the staffing hierarchy, changes in administrative procedures, and practitioners would be expected to "work with poor people, to do therapy under observation where all errors are visible and quite possibly have the results of their therapy evaluated"; there would also be "service to larger numbers of people, less of a waiting list, more time devoted to therapy . . . and better treatment outcome" (p. 12). Haley offered managers and service organizers several ways to avoid family therapy interfering with their status quo. He suggested that managers could appear welcoming and interested in the approach at all times while doing nothing to facilitate family therapy services, in the hope that practitioners enthusiastic about family therapy would eventually lose interest. Alternatively they could establish a family therapy section but find good reasons to avoid allocating it referrals, or they could refer the most difficult cases for family therapy while allocating the least experienced staff, untrained in the approach, to do the work.

I have met all of the above methods for avoiding family therapy and systemic practice in the course of my work with several different services. I have also come across a more extensive range of avoidant practices informed by the discourses of impossibility outlined above. This book represents examples of some exciting projects where the authors are using a systemic approach to create innovative and ethical services. They have *chosen* to ignore the voices of impossibility and have created an opportunity to share experiences of what *is possible*.

CHAPTER TWO

The use of the systemic approach to adults with intellectual disabilities and their families: historical overview and current research

Sandra Baum

Interest in applying the systemic approach through the methods and techniques of family therapy with adults with intellectual disabilities and their families has grown in the last ten years. This chapter examines what this approach has to offer. The chapter begins by defining the term "intellectual disabilities", documenting the evolution of this definition over time within the context of changing service provision. It then describes the models of the development of psychological services for people with intellectual disabilities within this context, highlighting the individualized focus of such services. A review is presented of the clinical and research literature concerning families where a member has intellectual disabilities, looking in turn at stress, coping, siblings, life-cycle transitions, loss, and parental patterns. Although much of the research described is not explicitly systemic in its focus, the paucity of systemic research with this client group means that this literature forms some useful evidence for those offering systemic family therapy to people with intellectual disabilities. Finally, the chapter examines the utility of family therapy with this client group; an example from practice is included to demonstrate the use of this model. It is concluded that although this approach has much to offer, appropriate ways of evaluating its theoretical ideas and therapy outcomes still need to be developed.

Definition of intellectual disabilities

The label "intellectual disabilities" is used to describe a heterogeneous group of people who have various degrees of intellectual and functional impairments compared to a norm. It is a socially constructed term, which means that how it is measured—and therefore who is counted as having "intellectual disabilities"—has varied over time (Wright & Digby, 1996). It is also defined differently cross-nationally according to cultural, political, economic, and ideological factors (Fryers, 1993). In the UK there have been many changes in the terminologies used over the last hundred years, which reflects different historical, philosophical, and cultural use of labels. These are discussed in what follows.

* * *

At the beginning of the twentieth century in the UK, the Mental Deficiency Act of 1913 was the first Act to supposedly give definitions of the various grades of "mental deficiency", which were restricted to those apparent from birth. It classified "defectives" under four headings: idiots, imbeciles, feebleminded persons, and moral defectives. These definitions were described in terms of "defects", rather than any scientific statement about what a defect is, and were for social and administrative purposes rather than clinical ones. They set the tone of that time, with the Eugenics Society in particular fearing a "national degeneracy" resulting from the "propagation of the unfit" (Race, 1995, p. 16), which was the impetus towards the segregation of people with intellectual disabilities (discussed further in the next section). However, these were the legal categories for nearly half a century afterwards.

* * *

Also around that time in France and the USA, the notion of a "scientific" classification of the development of mind was gaining momentum. In 1911, Binet and Simon published tests that focused on the underlying idea that "mental age" was related to chronological age and that this could provide an "intelligence quotient" (IQ). Thus, mental ability was seen as a physiological function unchanging over time, which could be measured scientifically by standardized methods. Although

IQ classification has long been criticized and debated (Race, 1995), it continues to be widely used as one of the primary ways of defining "intellectual disabilities".

* * *

The term "mental handicap" grew in popularity after the publication of the government White Paper *Better Services for the Mentally Handicapped* (Department of Health & Social Security [DHSS], 1971) and with the growth of a greater variety of services and non-medical staff caring for people with intellectual disabilities (Race, 1995). In the UK, "learning disabilities" was introduced by the Department of Health to replace "mental handicap" in 1992, and this is the term most commonly used in the UK (Department of Health, 1992). A person is considered to have learning disabilities if she or he has both impairments of cognitive and social functioning and these have been present since before the age of 18 years (American Association on Mental Retardation, 2002). The commonly accepted definition relies on an IQ measurement of 2 standard deviations below the population mean (IQ 69 or less) (British Psychological Society, 2001). This has to be accompanied by substantial limitations in present functioning and adaptive skills such as self-care and social skills (American Association on Mental Retardation, 2002).

* * *

Internationally, the term "intellectual disabilities" is becoming more widely used in order to reduce confusion as to which client group is being referred to. This is the term that is used in this book (the rationale for using this term is explained in the Introduction). Alternative terminologies may be used when quoting from the wider literature. Changing historical, political, and social contexts are continually modifying the definition of intellectual disabilities, and a precise definition is the subject of endless debate (Danforth & Navaro, 1998). People with intellectual disabilities come into contact with professional services for a wide variety of reasons, such as behavioural, emotional, and life-cycle issues. Thus, the psychology of intellectual disabilities is the interaction between the disability (the organic impairment) and society's response to it (Clements, 1987; Hennicke, 1993).

Services for people with intellectual disabilities

Changing service models

The definition of intellectual disabilities has changed over time, along with changes in services and philosophies of care. In the late-nineteenth and early twentieth centuries, service models tended to be medicalized, with the routine hospitalization and segregation of people with intellectual disabilities. Since the 1970s, service models have become more individualized in their philosophies but have rarely explicitly considered systemic models (McIntosh, 2002). Until relatively recently there have also been general limitations in services to address the emotional needs of people with intellectual disabilities (Arthur, 1999). In the following sections the history, development, and current climate of services in the UK will be described, as these form the context for the development of the systemic approach and family therapy services for adults with intellectual disabilities and their families.

The early twentieth century

In the early twentieth century, people with intellectual disabilities were considered something of a threat to society for two main and overlapping reasons. First, the medical profession became very influential and began to propose that "idiocy" was an organic disease that could not be cured. This contributed to the notion that people with intellectual disabilities were qualitatively different from the rest of society. Second, the eugenics movement feared that the national gene pool was at risk from those at the lower end of the social scale. In particular, this applied to women with intellectual disabilities (defined as "feeble-minded"), who were thought to be promiscuous, immoral, and likely to produce large numbers of children like themselves due to excessive fertility (Fernald, 1893). Both men and women with intellectual disabilities were seen as having very strong sexual inclinations, coupled with poor personal control, "making them a menace to society at large" (Craft, 1987, p. 14). This idea led to people with intellectual disabilities being routinely institutionalized and segregated to prevent reproduction, perhaps even compulsorily sterilized (the latter more common in the USA than in the UK: Barker, 1983) to ensure that inferior genes could not be passed on to future generations. The permanent segregation of people with a "mental deficiency" was thus an explicit goal for institutions (Jackson, 1996).

The 1970s

In the latter half of the twentieth century, the situation started to change in the UK. Research began to show that the institutions had debilitating effects, with barren environments offering little education or the teaching of skills. There were also a series of scandals concerning hospitals for people with intellectual disabilities, starting with Ely Hospital in 1969 (see Race, 1995), which highlighted how hospital staff ill-treated their patients. As a consequence, in recognition of the growing awareness of the negative effects of institutionalization, the 1971 White Paper *Better Services for the Mentally Handicapped* (Department of Health & Social Security, 1971) and the 1979 Jay Report (Jay, 1979) both recommended closing down hospitals and developing community-based services.

The 1980s and 1990s

In the 1980s and 1990s many of the institutions closed, and the ideology of "normalization" (Wolfensberger, 1972; re-termed "social role valorization" by Wolfensberger in 1983), gained enormous impact on attitudes and services. The normalization concept originated first in Denmark and Scandinavia (Bank-Mikkelsen, 1980; Nirje, 1980) and went on to be developed in North America (Wolfensberger, 1972, 1983). In Britain, the five service accomplishments of choice, community presence, community participation, competence, and respect (O'Brien, 1987) have also been influential. These operationalized the principles of normalization. Normalization states that it is society that disables people by the limited and devalued experiences it offers and that the way to overcome this is to increase people's social status. It has resulted in the increasing recognition of the right of people with intellectual disabilities to receive community care and to lead ordinary lives in their local communities. The effect has been to increase community housing and access to ordinary social and health services, including a range of psychological and therapeutic services that had been limited in the past. Normalization has been criticized from both feminist and race/ethnicity perspectives (e.g., see Brown & Smith, 1989, 1992; Ferns, 1992). It has also been argued that service provision is still falling short of "ordinary" life principles in many areas (Mental Health Foundation, 1996). In spite of this there is a consensus that it has been immensely valuable in improving the lives of millions of people with intellectual disabilities (McCarthy, 1999).

* * *

The advocacy movement also started to develop in the 1980s and 1990s and had many achievements such as the growth of self-advocacy (e.g., see Simons, 1992). Its aim was to empower people to understand their rights and to communicate them effectively to others. This has influenced many current service developments, such as the growth in supported living, supported employment, and changing day-service provision (Mental Health Foundation, 1996). However, services have by and large been slow to respond. It has been argued that this is "due to the usual reluctance of those in power to relinquish it" (McCarthy, 1999, p. 48). Whether this is right or not, there is no doubt that the movement, although irreversible, has developed unevenly but will continue to grow in influence.

The twenty-first century

The most recent English White Paper, *Valuing People: A New Strategy for Learning Disability for the 21st Century* (Department of Health, 2001) and the counterparts in Scotland, *The Same as You? A Review of Services for People with Learning Disabilities* (Scottish Executive, 2000), and Wales, *Fulfilling the Promises: Proposal for a Framework for Services for People with Learning Disability* (Learning Disability Advisory Group, 2001), further emphasized the principles of rights, independence, choice, and inclusion originally targeted in the concept of normalization. These White Papers cover every aspect of the lives of people with intellectual disabilities. The main focus is to give people with intellectual disabilities and their parents or carers more choice and control over their lives and the services and support they receive, primarily through a person-centred approach. The White Papers also state that the planning and delivery of services for people with intellectual disabilities should be included in the planning of services for all other members of the community, so that social inclusion is a reality for all.

Psychological services

Most psychological services for people with intellectual disabilities developed in the 1960s and 1970s, when behaviourism was the predominant psychological model. This model stated that all behaviour was triggered by environmental events or maintained by the consequences of behaving in a particular way. The behavioural approach (Yule & Carr, 1980; La Vigna & Donnellan, 1986) shaped the nature of interventions developed for people with intellectual disabilities and their carers (Caine, Hatton, & Emerson, 1998). During the 1980s, the hardline behaviourism of the 1960s and 1970s gradually developed into a more ethical behavioural approach, which considered the individual needs, rights, and wishes of the person with intellectual disabilities. Through concentrating on the interaction between the individual and their environment by using a "functional analysis" (Owens & Ashcroft, 1982)—that is, analysing the "function" of the problem or symptom for the individual—consideration was given to the emotional and cognitive aspects of behaviour (Zarkowska & Clements, 1988).

* * *

In the late 1980s and 1990s, the influence of normalization led to the development of a range of client-focused therapies to address the emotional and mental health difficulties of people with intellectual disabilities. Cognitive behavioural models (see Stenfert Kroese, Dagnan, & Loumidis, 1997) and psychotherapeutic models (see Sinason, 1992; Beail, 1995) gained acceptance in psychological services. (Cognitive behavioural models take into consideration the individual's thoughts and assumptions and argue that these will affect overt behaviour as well as emotions. Psychotherapeutic models concentrate on the individual's internal world and early experiences.) Despite this changing philosophical picture, for many people with intellectual disabilities, most of their basic mental health needs were traditionally forgotten or denied by services—for example, they rarely had someone to listen to them and help make sense of important events—though the need for such services was evident (Sinason, 1992; Bender, 1993; Wright & Digby, 1996; Gardner & Rikberg Smyly, 1997; Arthur, 1999). It is still the case today across Britain that the provision of psychotherapeutic services offered to this client group remains patchy.

In summary, psychological services have been slow to respond to the emotional needs of people with intellectual disabilities. It is perhaps, therefore, unsurprising that they have also been slow to respond to the emotional needs of the families and carers of people with intellectual disabilities. These individualized approaches may have further contributed to the lack of family-based services, including the use of systemic approaches. In other UK contexts, such as child and family services, systemic approaches—primarily family therapy—have traditionally been used with families presenting with a range of issues and have been shown to have positive effects. Positive changes have been documented in the symptoms of the named client and in family interactions when compared with alternative interventions or no intervention (e.g., Carr, 1991; Brent et al., 1997; Jones & Asen, 2000). These findings suggest that this approach could also be useful for people with intellectual disabilities and their families. This is discussed further later in this chapter.

Families of people with intellectual disabilities

The preceding discussion highlights the limitations of services in addressing the emotional needs of both people with intellectual disabilities and their families and carers. It also describes the development of individualized service philosophies, which have tended to medicalize or pathologize the person with intellectual disabilities, seeing his or her problems as inherent to the person: they have been mainly deficit-based, thus ignoring people's resources and abilities, and have often been a-contextual. In contrast, what is distinct about the systemic approach is its central emphasis on context and relational aspects of people's lives. As the Kensington Consultation Centre (2004) underlines: "The systemic approach explores the networks of significant relationships of which each individual is a part, considering the beliefs that give meaning to people's actions and the communication patterns between people as they interact with each other and with each other's ideas"(p. 4).

Of course, in this context the systemic approach must include not just families but also a wider network of other people. Some people with intellectual disabilities do not live with their families, some are estranged from their families, and some live in residential homes or in supported living accommodation. There will usually also be carers (paid or unpaid), extended family members, a GP, and other professionals—for example, the community team for people with intellectual disabilities, social services, and voluntary agencies. A close look at the interaction between the person with intellectual disabilities, the family system where relevant, and the various external support systems is crucial when working within a systemic approach.

* * *

This section reviews the general family research in intellectual disabilities; the subsequent sections highlight themes that are relevant to a systemic approach, emphasizing its usefulness for this client group and their families. Much of the family research described is not explicitly systemic in its focus, but it can be used as a source of knowledge to draw on by those offering systemic family therapy to people with intellectual disabilities. Although this section does not focus on those people who live in residential homes and their paid carers, similar themes may equally apply to the interactions of these subsystems. These interactions are explored further by Selma Rikberg Smyly in her chapter on working with staff teams (chapter eight).

Family research in intellectual disabilities: a review

Family-based care has always has been one of the dominant residential arrangements for people with intellectual disabilities (Seltzer, 1992) in spite of the large numbers of people who were institutionalized from the early twentieth century (Race, 1995). The lifespan of people with intellectual disabilities now approximates to that of the general population (Grant, 1990). This means that more and more people with intellectual disabilities are living with, or actually outliving, their ageing parents (Seltzer, 1992). Nevertheless, most of the family research in intellectual disabilities has focused on young children and their parents (Blacher, 1984; Byrne & Cunningham, 1985), and, until recently, scant attention was paid to the families of adults with intellectual disabilities. Most of the research is not from a systemic perspective; however, it is relevant in providing background knowledge of issues particularly pertinent to these families. The existing literature highlights three themes: stress, coping and siblings. These are examined here in turn.

Stress

Initial work concerning families who have a young child with intellectual disabilities (e.g., Evans & Carter, 1954; Kew, 1975) adopted a pathological approach that made the assumption that such families were inevitably subject to high levels of stress. These studies suffered from methodological problems because of assuming homogeneity among their sample groups. Later approaches became more sophisticated (e.g., Crnic, Friedrich, & Greenberg, 1983; Byrne & Cunningham, 1985; Seligman & Darling, 1989). They considered the structure of the family unit, relationships within the family, stressors, and the material, psychological, and social resources available to the family as potential contributors to the process of coping, rather than assuming that these families would be necessarily subject to high levels of stress. Byrne and Cunningham (1985) argued that stress for individual family members will change over time and that not all parents of children with intellectual disabilities would experience high levels of stress all the time.

* * *

Research on vulnerability factors related to the stresses of caring for a person with intellectual disabilities has highlighted the characteristics of that adult (diagnosis; physical health; level of behavioural problems; severity of intellectual disabilities; and physical dependence) as well as parental characteristics such as financial difficulties, marital problems, and social isolation (see Seltzer & Krauss, 1989; Grant & McGrath, 1990; Greenberg, Seltzer, & Greenley, 1993). Unmet local service needs are also associated with stress for many parents (Byrne & Cunningham, 1985; Roccoforte, 1991), as well as the lack of a coordinated approach that considers the needs of the whole family (Mitchell & Sloper, 2000).

Coping

Research has also looked at families who cope. It has attempted to specify factors that facilitate coping, including social-support networks; marital satisfaction; physical health and emotional well-being within the family; positive problem-solving skills; high income; and the family's social climate, ideological beliefs, and perceptions (see Folkman, Schaefer, & Lazarus, 1979; Crnic, Friedrich, & Greenberg, 1983; Kazak & Martin, 1984; Fatimilehin & Nadirshaw, 1994).

Siblings

There is a small literature on siblings that argues that an extra burden may be placed on the non-disabled siblings, because they may be asked to assume an adult role. Gath (1973) found that siblings revealed a higher incidence of behavioural problems. Cleveland and Miller (1977) found that the heaviest demands were placed on older sisters. Gath and Gumley (1987), however, did not replicate these findings. Shulman (1988) presented two examples from practice which suggested that parents may develop coping strategies, aimed at responding to the needs of the child with intellectual disabilities, that may hamper the development of the well siblings. However, negative consequences are by no means the norm. Reactions may change over time and will be influenced by interpretations and understandings of disability, together with the degree of support available from parents and others outside the family (Bromley, 1998).

Summary

Because most of the family-based care research in intellectual disabilities has focused on young children and their parents, it is difficult to generalize these findings to adults with intellectual disabilities and their parents. Some of the main criticisms of the research are that it has tended to focus on mothers only. Vetere (1993) notes that, as a result of this, there has been little attempt at directly observing family life and thus there is "a lack of a unified family research model" (p. 116). There is scant literature on the role of fathers (Seligman & Darling, 1989), and this is an area where research is urgently needed. There are also few studies that look at adults living with family members throughout their lives or that focus on the cumulative effects that caring for longer than three or four decades has on ageing parents.

* * *

Some of the existing research, though, has relevance in providing a historical context when working systemically with adults with intellectual disabilities and their families. For example, patterns and interactions that may have been established in the earlier years of the child's life are likely to continue and perhaps influence adult relationships. Some of these issues are discussed in the next section.

Themes relevant to a systemic approach

In the family research and systemic literature, there are a number of predominant themes that have been shown to impact on families of young children with intellectual disabilities, and, more recently, families of adults with intellectual disabilities, that are relevant to working systemically. These themes may change in their emotional intensity according to the current family situation and problems, but they provide clues as to how the family communicates, interacts, and relates and may guide therapists' hypotheses about presenting problems. These themes include transitions and the family life-cycle; patterns such as the concept of "perpetual parents"; and relationships with wider systems.

Transitions and the family life-cycle

Issues of transition have been written about extensively in the intellectual disabilities literature, but this has rarely used a systemic frame. One useful model that has been applied is the family life-cycle (Carter & McGoldrick, 1989). Concepts relevant in the intellectual disabilities field such as "out of synchrony", grief, loss, and protection have particular resonance when applied to this model.

"Family life-cycle" theory focuses on the family moving through time rather than on specific family members. Carter and McGoldrick (1989) described a sequence of life-cycle transitions that create stressors within the family system as individuals reorganize and negotiate change, such as the birth of a child, going to school, leaving home, family illness, and death. Their theory considered how stressors such as family patterns, myths and secrets, and legacies can facilitate or hinder the process of transition. Transitions can upset the homeostasis of the family because they often demand a change in how the family interacts and disturb its previous behaviour patterns. How families cope at different stages will depend on what life-cycle issues each member faces at that time. For example, an adult with intellectual disabilities may want to move out of the home to become more independent at the very time that a parent desires companionship, perhaps because of widowhood. A family member may become "symptomatic" if the family cannot adapt or negotiate this new transition.

"Out of synchrony"

One central issue for families who have an intellectually disabled member is that the sequence of life events is often different to that experienced by families without disabilities (Vetere, 1993). Transitions may be "arrested" or appear "out of synchrony" in families with a disabled member (Goldberg et al., 1995). For example, adults with intellectual disabilities who live with their parents for much of their adult life are often faced with their first transition out of the family home rather late in life, after their parents die or become ill. (This stage usually occurs after other life-cycle events have run their course.)

Grief and loss

A second central issue is the concept of "chronic sorrow" (Wikler, Waslow, & Hatfield, 1981). In Wikler et al.'s study, parents described how "chronic sorrow" or disappointment emerged in the family at various transition points in a child with intellectual disabilities' life. Family members are faced with the loss of previously held expectations as the person fails to conform to the cultural norms of family development. In her seminal paper of 1983, Bicknell expanded on this idea. Life events in the family—even those that have nothing to do with the disabled child—can bring up issues of unresolved loss and grief "for the perfect child who has not arrived" (Bicknell, 1983, p. 168). Goldberg et al. (1995) argued that difficulties at different life-cycle stages may act as a painful reminder of this grief and noted that feelings of loss and anger may be re-evoked. In order to progress through the current transition, some families "may have to grieve their current losses, which will inevitably evoke a series of losses, each constrained by patterns of grieving for the losses that preceded them" (p. 269). Thus, the initial pattern of response to the original loss of hopes and expectations may be recapitulated at the next loss.

Protection

Linked to the evolving response to loss is the issue of "protection". Goldberg et al. (1995) argue that families that include a person with intellectual disabilities often have difficulties progressing to the next life-cycle stage, such as the person with disabilities leaving home, because they want to protect that person from the perceived consequences of his or her disability. Protection often revolves around fear of violence, social and sexual activity, and death (Hollins & Grimer, 1988; Sinason, 1992). On the other hand, the family member with intellectual disabilities may protect his or her parents from the consequences of their old age and thoughts about their mortality by, for example, remaining at home and avoiding the grief of the "empty-nest" stage. In other words, family members together may avoid life-cycle transitions such as leaving home and therefore further loss. Often families seek help from services when this protection is either failing or is counterproductive (Goldberg et al., 1995).

* * *

The life-cycle framework aids understanding of the difficulties of particular families, their potential stresses, their crisis points, and their reactions and needs. It also helps us to consider why a family may have presented for help to services at a particular point. Clearly, though, there are limitations with stage models. Parents' responses to their child's disability are very individual and will be greatly influenced by their own beliefs, the extended family's views on disability, together with societal and cultural beliefs and constructions. Conversely, many young people do not follow a normative route of leaving home in their late teens or early twenties but may stay considerably longer, and thus their parents may face similar struggles to those whose children have intellectual disabilities.

Parental patterns

Studying parents of co-residing adult offspring with intellectual disabilities, Todd and Shearn (1996) identified two groups of parents of adults with intellectual disabilities whom they named "perpetual parents". The first were "captive parents" or "perpetual parents in the making" who found living a "normal life" increasingly difficult and experienced a sense of loss associated with this. The second were "captivated parents", who were committed to their parenting lifestyles because losing their parenting role would be a significant loss of self-meaning and would be difficult to replace. Although this research is not from the systemic literature, it is useful because it provides insight into why it may be difficult for some families to enable their adult offspring to become more independent if it means relinquishing their caring role. The main problem with this research is that it assumes a dichotomy between the two groups. It is possible that parents oscillate between these two states at different times in their lives.

Relationship with wider systems

The interactions between the person with intellectual disabilities, his or her family, and wider systems are complex. Many alliances and coalitions are possible, as well as many differences of opinion and perception. These may be related to educational issues; the nature of the disability and its likely response to treatment; the aetiology and maintenance of behavioural difficulties; and what options there are for the future (in terms of placement, daytime activities, independence, etc.). The family will have its own historical context, which may have evolved out of its experience with services in the past. The way in which these systems interact with the family may affect how they present for help to services and will also affect engagement, expectations, and possible solutions to crises. These issues are clearly vital to consider in any therapeutic interaction (for further discussion of these issues, see Hennicke, 1993; Goldberg et al., 1995).

* * *

Various authors have elaborated on these themes. Imber-Black (1987) suggests that the individual with intellectual disabilities interacts with both family and "human delivery" systems. Change at one level may not be mirrored elsewhere, causing disequilibrium and conflict and thus uncertainty for families and professionals alike. Stressors are particularly likely at family life-cycle transitions, when comparisons between intellectually disabled and non-disabled peers tend to become manifest (Seligman & Darling, 1989; Vetere, 1993; Evans & Midence, 1999). In this situation, interventions must necessarily take into account the characteristics of each overlapping system (Dale, 1995; Bromley, 1998). Clegg (1993) further develops this perspective by suggesting the need to examine four system levels—intrapersonal, interpersonal, positional, and ideological—and argues that a social constructionist framework may provide the best way of conceptualizing these together.

Family therapy with adults with intellectual disabilities and their families

Interest in using systemic approaches in working with people with intellectual disabilities and their families has grown since the 1980s. Turner (1980), Black (1987), Shulman (1988), Roy-Chowdhury (1992), Hennicke (1993), and Cobb and Gunn (1994) all give examples where family therapy has been effective with children and their families. Thomson (1986), Vetere (1993), Goldberg et al. (1995), Fidell (1996, 2000), Salmon (1996), Baum, Chapman, Scior, Sheppard, and Walden (2001), and Lynggaard and Scior (2002) have presented accounts of their work involving adults with intellectual disabilities that suggest that systemic interventions may be helpful for this client group. In addition, Dixon and Matthews (1992) have shown that teaching family therapy techniques to community nurses working with adults with intellectual disabilities and their families can enhance their skills in managing difficult situations by making them "more aware of the complexity and difficulty of the situations they are dealing with" (p. 17).

The usefulness of family therapy in this area

The systemic approach may offer a number of advantages over individually focused interventions. First, as we have seen, there is some evidence of higher emotional stress for many families at life-cycle transitions which may be exacerbated by the experience of discrimination and blame (Turnbull, Summers, & Brotherson, 1986; Fidell, 2000). These difficulties may be more appropriately addressed through family therapy, because it considers life-cycle and power issues as integral. Second, as has also been described, there are often concerns about the interaction with the wider care system (Fidell, 2000). Families are frequently involved with numerous services, which can blur the boundaries between parental and agency responsibility (Vetere, 1993). The systemic approach can be useful in negotiating the complexity of relationships and communications between different sub-systems which can be confusing for family members (Mitchell & Sloper, 2000). It is also significant that, when asked about service provision, families often say that they would favour a coordinated approach that takes into consideration the needs of the whole family (Mitchell & Sloper, 2000). Finally, the systemic approach seeks to understand concerns, problems, or difficulties within the contexts in which they emerge and in the context of relationships.

Including the person with intellectual disabilities in family therapy

Adaptations of systemic family therapy may be necessary to meet the needs of the person with intellectual disabilities. Many practitioners have described adaptations to enable the engagement of the person with intellectual disabilities such as specific therapeutic skills and techniques to concretize the therapeutic process and aim for a slower therapeutic pace (e.g., see Goldberg et al., 1995; Fidell, 1996, 2000; Salmon, 1996; Lynggaard & Scior, 2002). An example of this is provided by Fidell (1996). She describes "circular showing" (Benson, Schindler-Zimmerman, & Martin, 1991, cited in Fidell, 1996), as an adaptation to circular questioning (i.e., the ability to step outside a given relationship and observe it in operation). By simplifying the way relationship questions are put to people with intellectual disabilities using role-plays, drawings, symbols, and visual aids, the disabled person can be included in the interaction, as these techniques reduce the cognitive demands of relational dialogues. Bromley (1998) also states that asking certain questions of *all* family members in each other's presence may give clues as to how the person with disabilities is included in the family, in terms of how people respond and communicate with that person, who advocates for whom, and so forth. These ideas are further elaborated in chapters five and ten.

Raena and Meena

The following example highlights some of the themes discussed that might benefit from being addressed by family therapy.

Raena and Meena were two sisters who were initially both referred to the community health team for people with intellectual disabilities for family therapy by their social worker because the sisters hit each other and because the eldest, Raena, hit her mother too. This behaviour had escalated in the last year. Raena went to a local day centre, and Meena was in the final year of a special school for children with intellectual disabilities.

Raena and Meena were 21 and 19 years old, with mild and severe intellectual disabilities, respectively. They lived with their parents, Mr and Mrs Pathwa, who were originally from Pakistan but had lived in the UK for twenty-three years. Both parents had extended families but said that they did not get any support from them. Meena was on high levels of medication due to her epilepsy and had to attend frequent hospital appointments. In the first family therapy session, Mr and Mrs Pathwa said that doctors had told them that neither child would survive into adulthood as both had a degenerative disease. This diagnosis was changed when the children were 7 and 5 years, respectively, with the doctors now asserting that a genetic link had caused their disabilities. Neither parent wanted to know which side of the family was to "blame". Both parents also reported that if they argued in either of their daughters' presence, this would often lead to Raena hitting her sister or mother. Both parents would then separate them, and each would spend time with one of their daughters in order to stop them fighting.

* * *

Within intellectual disability services, a referral such as this could have been approached from an individualized perspective, locating the problem of the hitting behaviour within Raena and Meena themselves. Interventions such as introducing medication, using behaviour modification, or concentrating on their internal worlds and early experiences by offering psychodynamic psychotherapy could have been employed in an attempt to help reduce the problem behaviour. A systemic approach, with its emphasis on relationships, shifts the focus from the person in isolation to the person in context and posits that people both influence, and are influenced by, the systems within which they interact. In this example, several factors encouraged us to use a systemic perspective. Raena had already been seen by a clinical psychologist a year before for problems around hitting her mother, and a behavioural approach had been employed, but with only limited success. There was evidence of relational difficulties within the family. And finally, the mother and father wanted to be seen as a family because they both said that their daughters' behaviour affected them all.

* * *

It was hypothesized with the family that the triggering event that led to an escalation of difficulties was both children's life-cycle transition from childhood to adulthood. For Raena and Meena, leaving school marked a new definition for them in the family—that is, a change from child to adult. However, the fact that both daughters were intellectually disabled and would still be dependent on their parents reinforced the perception that they were children rather than young adults.

* * *

Linked with this hypothesis was the concept of "chronic sorrow". Mr and Mrs Pathwa both talked about the early years of their children's lives and had feelings of guilt and shame. Whose "fault" was it that the children were born disabled? These feelings had not been aired or shared between them, possibly resulting in marital difficulties. It was hypothesized that the daughters' hitting behaviour may have developed because of communication problems between the parents. The behaviour served the homeostatic function of detouring the parents' tension—that is, who was to blame for their disabilities—as they both found it hard to talk about their feelings, which increased the distance between them as a couple. The hitting behaviour also had the function of uniting the parents in a shared task—that of parenting—as opposed to arguing, which might potentially separate them.

* * *

In this example, the goals of therapy agreed with the family included exploring with Mr and Mrs Pathwa the meanings and beliefs they attributed to living with two disabled daughters and the impact that it might have on them as a couple. (These discussions took place without their daughters joining them in the session, as it felt important to offer the parents a space to talk about some of the issues and feelings identified above.) Another goal was to enable them to discriminate between parental and marital tensions and the way they interacted with each other and their daughters. Discussion focused on their angry feelings towards their extended families, who were unsupportive and ignored their children. Mr and Mrs Pathwa had different ways of showing and coping with these feelings, which led to tension between them. The sessions were also used to discuss their daughters' difficult behaviour, taking into account the family interactions by exploring how to accommodate their different understandings rather than them being detoured through their daughters. Discussion also focused on the issues of dependence, independence, and interdependence now that both daughters had reached the life-cycle transition of adolescence to adulthood.

* * *

The family was seen for ten sessions over seventeen months (three of these sessions were attended by the parents alone). The outcome was that Mr and Mrs Pathwa reported that they were not arguing as much, and their children were not hitting each other as much. Both parents had become aware of how focusing just on their daughters' "difficult" behaviour had prevented them from discussing the meanings and beliefs they had about Raena and Meena becoming adults and how this transition in turn brought up feelings of grief.

* * *

It was very difficult to engage Raena and Meena fully in the work. However, they were very much part of the process and were invited to be present while their parents talked about some of their own difficulties. Fidell (2000) argues that this must be a novel experience, as many people with intellectual disabilities "hear themselves being talked about much of the time and were not supposed to listen" (p. 315). Also, if the hitting behaviour was an expression of a fear that the parents might separate, then it was less necessary for the young women to always be in the foreground, as they had succeeded in bringing the parents together to address some of the issues that were of concern.

Conclusions

The application of systemic ideas and principles in working with families of adults with intellectual disabilities, particularly using family therapy, is an exciting and innovative development. Clements (1992) discusses the advantages of applying the findings from mainstream psychological literature to this client group and argues that it contributes to the social valuation of people with intellectual disabilities, since it emphasizes "a perception of their commonalties with, rather than their differences from, other people in society" (p. 30).

* * *

The widespread neglect of systemic issues, which has often characterized psychological work with adults with intellectual disabilities, can be at least partly attributed to three factors. First, until recently scant attention was paid to families of adults with intellectual disabilities, with most research focusing instead on the needs of young children with intellectual disabilities and their parents. Second, the systemic literature has paid little attention to the needs of families with an intellectually disabled member. Third, psychological services for people with intellectual disabilities have tended to focus on individual approaches rather than viewing the person in his or her wider context. The small number of studies that have been published have illustrated that this approach can be very useful in efforts to understand and respond to the difficulties that adults with intellectual disabilities and their families may face. Undoubtedly, systemic approaches to working with this client group are very much in their infancy, and we have much to learn about models and, above all, creative approaches to working systemically with clients who often lack sufficient communication skills to make use of "standard" systemic techniques.

* * *

As the systemic approach gains popularity among practitioners working with people with intellectual disabilities, we will need to reflect on our own and our clients' experiences of this work through single case studies. We will also need to find appropriate ways of evaluating theoretical ideas and therapy outcomes through larger-scale empirical studies. The themes highlighted in this chapter pose very fruitful questions for research, particularly as it is becoming increasingly accepted that the systemic approach may have much to offer to work with people with intellectual disabilities.

CHAPTER THREE

Lifespan family therapy services

Sabrina Halliday and Lorna Robbins

When the Leeds Family Psychology and Therapy Service (Leeds FPTS) was set up in 1995, the principles of choice and inclusion were paramount. We wanted to offer the choice of a family therapy service to those people and their families, partners, or carers who traditionally would not have easy access to this form of therapy. We believed that older adults and their families, people with intellectual disabilities and those they lived with, and adults with serious mental health problems could benefit from family therapy. We also questioned the need to have separate child and adult teams. We wanted to provide a family service across the lifespan and draw practitioners from all clinical specialities. This would increase the pool of practitioners available. It would also facilitate access to specialized services for family members where other care needs were identified.

* * *

The Leeds FPTS functions as a tertiary service. Referrals follow a comprehensive mental health needs assessment at the secondary level (Leeds FPTS, 2002). For example, the community team would constitute a secondary-level service for adults with intellectual disabilities. A community nurse might assess that a young man with intellectual disabilities requires individual work regarding his sexuality (which the nurse will provide) and additional family work to help prepare for the move from home. Family therapy, therefore, forms a component in a wider package of care. If the service-user chooses family therapy, there are no other eligibility criteria to meet.

The aims of this chapter

The key aim of this chapter, discussed in the first section, is to describe the way that the Leeds FPTS developed and works. In the second section we explore lifespan working. We consider how the lifespan approach provides a unique perspective on systemic working in general, and how the broader resources of the lifespan team are more able to open up the resources of the family and extended-care systems. In the third section we have provided a fairly long example to illustrate how we typically work with people with intellectual disabilities and their network. In the fourth section we provide the feedback and reflections of the clients and carers on their involvement in systemic therapy (and some of the learning points their comments have generated for us). We have also consulted with the practitioners in the service who do not specialize in working with people with intellectual disabilities; their comments on offering a systemic therapy service to people with intellectual disabilities are set out in the fifth section. We conclude the chapter by summarizing what have been some of the key learning points for us in establishing and running a lifespan service.

The development of the lifespan service

The service developed from a small group of practitioners, interested in family working, who noted an absence of family therapy services, particularly for devalued groups. The idea of a lifespan service initially began to form after a secretary working across child-and-adult specialities noticed members of the same family being referred to different therapeutic services. There followed two years of planning (1993–1995), with the eventual submission of a business plan. From the outset, the principles of choice, inclusion, equality, and accessibility across the lifespan were prioritized. The idea of a lifespan service was unique among the predominately child-oriented family services available within Leeds. A survey of potential referrers, GPs, and secondary services was conducted to predict referral rates to a city-wide lifespan family therapy service. This survey clearly established a demand among referrers and general enthusiasm for a lifespan approach.

* * *

After negotiating room-space in a central location, and gaining an informal agreement that practitioners could allocate one session a week to this work, the service opened in 1995. As a result, practitioners from different professions and backgrounds came together to form the team and co-author its evolving culture. The team is able to see two families a week in its afternoon clinic. Families attend for, on average, three sessions, at approximately monthly intervals (Leeds FPTS, 2002). When referral rates are high, we are fortunate to have the flexibility to add in an extra session. As a result of gradual expansion and training placements, two clinic teams were created. Between the two clinic sessions, both teams meet together for supervision. We also discuss research and theoretical ideas that relate to the families currently being seen.

* * *

We wanted to reflect further on our practice and evaluate our work. From 1997 onwards, trainee clinical psychologists were helpful in undertaking service-orientated research projects. For example, Hailstone (1997) looked at family satisfaction with the service. She found that families who had experienced both a Milan message (where the lead practitioner returned to the family towards the end of the session with a brief summary of the views of the team behind the one-way mirror) and, on another occasion, the reflecting-team method (where the team behind the one-way mirror swapped places with the family, so that the family could observe the team's reflecting conversation), preferred the reflecting team. Ingram (2000), from her participant observation in the teams over a period of a year, drew together nine emergent principles that appeared to guide the team's work. These are listed in Table 3.1. We have subsequently found her summary useful when describing our way of working to other teams or to people interested in joining our team.

Table 3.1. The nine guiding principles of the Leeds Family Psychology and Therapy Service (Ingram, 2000)

1. The focus is on the family as a system rather than on an individual.
2. Family and systemic therapy practice is considered a shared process.
3. While acknowledging problems and difficulties, the aim is not to pathologize people.
4. The team can facilitate the process of change by attending to families' strengths, resources, and abilities.
5. Times when problems are not influential in people's lives are identified and explored in order to understand and talk about what people do differently to subdue problems (cf. White, 1995).
6. The sessions provide a context in which family members can listen and talk to one another and feel able to express their opinions. Practitioners aim to facilitate this process.
7. The family and team work towards identifying specific goals that may provide a focus for the family sessions.
8. There may be multiple answers, explanations, or solutions to a given problem, and the family can choose which, if any, suits them or their circumstances.
9. The teams are respectful of the pace of therapy set by families: it is assumed that change can be hard work and cannot be forced or rushed.

Unique service approach

From the start, taking a lifespan perspective shaped the philosophy and practice of the service we aspired to provide. The essential elements of this philosophy are outlined below:

- *Integrated*—First, we view our approach as additional to and in collaboration with what the secondary service (i.e., the community team) is providing, not a replacement for it. Within the care package, family therapy may be the main element or it may be subsidiary. Second, the team is a resource, integrated with every part of the secondary health-care system, within the local Community Mental Health NHS Trust. Professionals in the team have their main work role within the secondary teams (e.g., intellectual disabilities, older adult, adult mental health, child and family, and forensic). We are able to integrate with different professional systems due to our different backgrounds. As a result, secondary teams are very aware of the work of the lifespan service and what is an appropriate referral. We have also connected with the carers and service-users group to develop information leaflets and to check the accessibility and "family-friendly feel" of the building. Third, we work across traditional "specialist" boundaries within the lifespan team, integrating our specialist knowledge within a systemic approach.

- *Inclusive*—From our experience, systemic therapy has something to offer everyone, and so the choice of participating in family therapy should be offered to all, whatever their age or ability. Being inclusive also means that different methods or models, which each team member uses to inform their thinking in systemic practice, are accepted within this approach. They are the seeds of multiple perspectives and provide the rich diversity of views that is essential for a team working with such a range of people. All of these enrich the team's ability to understand and recognize our own dominant narratives and constraints as well as our resources and voices (see Davidson, Lax, & Lussardi, 1990; Real, 1990; Lowe & Guy, 1996). We are constantly energized and inspired individually and, as a team, through our conversations with each other and with families.

- *Congruent*—The approach, methods, and techniques that we use with families are applied equally to ourselves. As a team we aim to use and develop effectively our strengths, resources, and abilities. We attempt to embrace multiple perspectives in our team, and we value curiosity, original ideas, experiences, as well as training. One way of doing this has been to use reflecting teams in supervision and training. We act as a training resource for our organization, including being a specialist placement for those in psychotherapy or clinical psychology training. We welcome all professionals who are interested in undertaking and applying systemic approaches within their practice, whatever their level of expertise. An agreed level of commitment to the team is required, so that families do not find that the composition of the team they see changes frequently. The minimum that we ask of the practitioner is that he or she follows one family through therapy and attends our weekly team meeting. New practitioners join as members of the reflecting team behind the one-way mirror. This reflects our belief that each of us has a valuable perspective to share. If practitioners are able to make a long-term commitment to the team, they may go on to take the role of lead practitioner with a family.

- *Ability discourse*—At many levels throughout a given system—cultural, legal, establishment, neighbourhood, friends, and family—dominant values tend to prescribe what is acceptable and worthy, and the converse: that which is unacceptable and worthless. Within a lifespan approach there are more opportunities to witness the numerous forms that a disability discourse may take. Most of the people who are referred to Leeds FPTS see their difficulties through these perspectives and feel stuck—for example, the child who is told and believes that he is a troublemaker and who is repeatedly excluded from school; the woman who views herself as a failure as a mother because she is at work when her children get home from school; the man who cannot see what he can offer his family since he lost his job; the couple who struggle with their family's view that their partnership is a burden to the woman since her husband had a stroke and so they ought to move to sheltered accommodation and give up their independent home. Working in a lifespan team makes these disabling discourses apparent across many families and groups, ages, and capacities. We have become aware of their influence, and they are more visible to us. Working systemically allows us to involve different parts of the system in addressing these discourses. Along with the families, we involve carers and other professionals as appropriate. We have found that change is facilitated when we can enable individuals and systems to become aware of their respective stories, strengths, and resources. This in turn enables each to question, and move away from, dominant problem-saturated stories.

The approach in practice

Our session structure is very similar to the way many family therapy teams practise in the UK, adopting a three-part format for the session (Lax, 1995). This comprises an interview between the lead practitioner and family (or other members of the system), a reflecting-team conversation in front of the family, and a post-reflection discussion between the lead practitioner and family. Our usual practice is to physically swap places during the reflection: the family and lead practitioner move behind the one-way mirror and the reflecting team move in front of it. After the reflection, we swap back.

* * *

In the following paragraphs, we describe what we think are the main elements of our practice that contribute to a shared, more constructive appreciation of what has been troubling to those who attend Leeds FPTS. We feel that our approach, with its emphasis on collaboration and non-pathologizing conversation, provides a distinctive experience for many families.

A systems focus

Rather than the person with intellectual disabilities being the "identified patient" where problems are located, we see the wider system as the "client". We work with immediate and extended family, direct-care staff, managers, other professionals, and other teams, depending on who the person and his or her immediate system see as influential in his or her problem. We acknowledge and recognize individual needs and joint struggles. We seek differing views on, and alternative stories to, the dominant narrative. We have found externalizing techniques a helpful way to do this (White & Epston, 1990a). The reflecting team often engages in conversations and observations that make the externalizations more explicit and, in the post-reflection conversation, may prompt "new knowledge" about relationships in the system.

A collaborative process

It is a working assumption made by the team that families are equipped with the ability to generate suitable solutions and the team is experienced in facilitating conversations that may be useful in achieving the family's identified goals for therapy (Tomm, 1989). We demonstrate our belief in the family's abilities by offering choice, for example, in the way the reflecting team is used and whether or not to make use of the one-way mirror. We work together, at a pace set by families, towards identifying a focus for the sessions. Towards the end of the post-reflection conversation, ideas about what the family might consider or do that have developed from the interplay of reflection and conversation about the reflection (co-constructed views) are discussed. People with intellectual disabilities have commented that having their ideas about what may work listened to is a new and positive experience. We adapt techniques to meet individual need—for example, we may use a summary letter or provide a video to aid recollection for people with intellectual disabilities (see also Fidell, 2000).

Recognizing resources

We look at the wider context of peoples' lives by being curious about skills and successes (Morgan, 1998). We explore times when problems are less evident or powerful and what people are doing differently. We ask who notices or encourages these positive times. The reflection includes recognition of both the concerns and strengths of family members and their efforts to find solutions. Team members make observations about occasions when the family has achieved positive outcomes and how this has been brought about and who their supporters are (George, Iveson, & Ratner, 1990; White, 1995).

Reflecting processes

There may be multiple answers, explanations, or solutions to a given problem or set of circumstances and the family can choose which, if any, suits them or their current situation. The techniques of reflection used by the team are based on Andersen's (1991) approach, summarized by Griffith and Elliott Griffith (1994), and focus on the variety of views and their contribution to the family story. The guidance of Bateson (1972) presenting "the difference that makes a difference" (p. 272) is borne in mind when tentatively offering another, slightly different viewpoint for consideration. The reflecting-team process allows each person the space to listen and to have an inner conversation with what they hear. In the post-reflection conversation they can reflect upon (outer conversation) what they have heard and what thoughts it generated. By active listening and discussing of other's perspectives (through inner and outer conversations), co-creation of an alternative or new understanding can take place (Andersen, 1987, 1991). These alternative, non-dominant narratives invariably include the family's strengths, resources and abilities, and ways of promoting them further.

Ruth and Wayne

The following example from our practice illustrates the flexible way that systemic approaches can be used to involve the significant people within the narrative at relevant times. It also confirms the ability of people with intellectual disabilities to participate fully in the systemic and reflecting processes, with appropriate attention to pacing and language. The example further illustrates many dominant themes in the lives of people with intellectual disabilities, particularly those of disempowerment and paternalism in relationships and life choices. The illustration is produced with the consent of the referred couple, with changes made to protect their identity but preserving the message of their story.

* * *

A brother and sister, in their mid-30s, both with intellectual disabilities, were referred to the team by their social worker. We were told that the couple had lived in their parental home until four years previously, when their father suffered an industrial injury, which necessitated the family moving to a smaller home and to their mother working part-time. As a result Ruth and Wayne moved to different flats within a local-authority hostel for adults with intellectual disabilities. At the time of the referral the small group flat in which Wayne lived was to be renovated, and it was proposed that Wayne should move permanently to another flat some five miles away. The referral was made because staff believed that the close relationship between Ruth and her brother was holding them both back from developing their potential. Staff wished the couple to receive counselling to enable them to separate and live independently. The Leeds FPTS agreed to see Ruth and Wayne and suggested that they decide whether they wished to come on their own or with staff.

First session: Ruth and Wayne arrived with their most trusted member of staff, Jim. We explained about the way the session could work, the presence of the reflecting team, confidentiality, and the use of the video for the team to reflect on sessions between appointments. Wayne and Ruth consented to be videoed, as did Jim, and said that they would like to have the reflecting team in the room for the reflection. The lead practitioner in the room (Colin) explained about the referral and asked them to tell us what they each thought it meant and what had brought them here.

Wayne: "Staff want us to be independent. I am going to live in the Crescent. I need to stand up for myself."

Colin (to Ruth): "What do you think when you hear Wayne say that?"

Ruth: "I'm sad already. I miss Wayne when he is away. I'm used to him being around."

Colin: "And why did you want to come and talk with us today?"

Ruth: "I'm sad."

Colin: "Did you know that your sister is sad about you moving to a new place?"

Wayne: "Ruth was sad when we moved away from home."

Ruth: "Yes, but I did not tell anyone then."

Wayne: "Ruth bottles things up."

Ruth: "Mmm."

Colin: "So, what happens when Ruth bottles things up?"

Wayne: "She goes pop!"

Colin: "She goes pop! What does Wayne mean by that, Ruth?"

Ruth: "I get very angry and I start shouting at Wayne and crying."

Wayne: "She shouts and I have to calm her down."

Colin: "Ruth bottles things up then she goes pop and you calm her down, and what do you do when you are upset or sad?"

Wayne: "I talk to Ruth, or Jim, staff and that helps."

Colin: "So you and Ruth do things differently and you also help each other, by listening to each other and calming each other down."

Wayne: "Ruth needs me to calm her down."

Colin: "So how will you help each other when you move to a new place, Wayne?"

Wayne: "I need to stand up for myself. I'm 34. I must learn to do things for myself. Jim says I will learn really fast when I live on my own."

Colin: "So you need to move to a new place where you can learn to do more things for yourself. That sounds quite exciting for you but it sounds sad for Ruth."

Wayne: "It's scary. Jim says it is scary too."

Colin: "Ruth, you are not sure what it will be like when Wayne moves away and you are not living together any more. Perhaps you find that a little scary too."

Ruth: "Yes, and yes a little scary when Wayne [sic] not with me."

Wayne: "Yes a little scary when Ruth and I will not live near together."

Ruth: "He will end up like I was, he will go pop."

In the remaining part of the session, Colin asked what they liked about living together and what they did now that they wanted to continue after the move. Some of the things they told us were that Ruth often did Wayne's shopping for him and that Wayne would lend Ruth money to go to the bingo. They occasionally went on the bus together to visit their parents.

* * *

During the reflection, one theme that emerged was about the big changes to Ruth's and Wayne's lives. The team were curious about their previous experiences of change (e.g., leaving their parents' home) and the resources they had drawn upon to cope in the past. Their skill in looking after themselves and each other was noted. "Closeness to family" was commented on as something very important in their lives. The team wondered: "What had they learned from their first big move that would be helpful now?" "How could they keep these special relationships when Wayne moved away to his new flat?" "Was there something special about being a brother and sister who had lived together for thirty years, which needed to be considered in their plans for the future?" The team also wondered: "How might Jim help them think about this?"

* * *

In the post-reflection, Wayne talked about how close they were as a family. He said he was worried about his dad dying. For her part, Ruth said that she missed the family and did not want Wayne to move away. Ruth was able to say this assertively rather than sadly. She said she felt safe when Wayne was nearby. This was a new element in the theme of closeness. It was one that Wayne seemed able to relate to. He put his arm around Ruth and said, "I will look after you".

* * *

Second session: Wayne and Ruth came by themselves to the second session. There it emerged that Wayne had already moved to his new flat because the renovation works had to start early. It became apparent that Wayne had been visiting Ruth almost every night and had to be asked to leave on several occasions so that the hostel could be locked up for the night. Ruth recalled, quite poignantly, that she could hear her brother's voice when he was not there, and this made her sad. Most of the session focused on how they were supporting each other through this difficult time.

Ruth: "I am helping Wayne get organized."

Wayne: "Yes, she is telling me what to do."

Ruth: "I worry about him."

Wayne: "You tell me off."

Ruth: "You have to do your shopping and you cannot come to the hostel when I am out at bingo!"

Colin: "Ruth, you seem to want to help Wayne get more settled in his new flat, you are helping him think about the things he has to do. Is that right?"

Ruth: "Yes, I am helping Wayne."

Colin: "Is that what is happening, Wayne?"

Wayne: "Yes, but I can come to the hostel to talk to staff."

Colin: "So sometimes Ruth helps you and sometimes you need the hostel staff to help you."

Wayne: "Mmm."

Ruth: "But they get fed up with him coming around all the time."

Colin: "What do you think?"

Ruth: "I like him to visit but I don't want him to get into trouble and shout at people."

Colin: "So you want Wayne to visit and Wayne wants to visit, but there can be arguments and shouting. What do you want Wayne?"

Wayne: "I need to stand up for myself and be independent."

The reflecting team commented upon how things had changed. Ruth felt more able to support Wayne in his move, but she also missed him and worried about him. Wayne wanted to visit his sister more, but he also wanted to learn how to live on his own. Perhaps this was causing tension for them both and creating arguments with staff. Members of the team wondered, "What it might be like in six months—would things be more settled?" "Would there be more arguments?" "What did Ruth want to be doing in six months' time?" In the post-reflection, Ruth and Wayne were asked to comment on what they had heard:

Post-reflection

Wayne: "You are spot on. I do need help, and I need to talk to staff and to Ruth to help me."

Ruth: "I want to help Wayne but I don't want him to get into trouble."

Colin: "So, how can you help each other?"

Ruth: "Maybe I can go round to Wayne's new flat sometimes."

Colin: "Have you been to his flat?"

Ruth: "No, I was too sad, but it will be OK now."

Colin: "Would that be helpful, Wayne?"

Wayne: "Yes, I would like Ruth to visit me—I tidy my flat."

By attending this session on their own, it seemed to free up Ruth and Wayne to discuss their own needs and the difficulties in their relationship in a more open and assertive way. The team's reflection on these difficulties, which put them in the context of their future, appeared to clarify for Wayne his view of himself as someone who would succeed at living alone, particularly if he could continue to get support from his sister and staff. Together Wayne and Ruth succeeded in finding a potential solution to adapting to living apart by agreeing to meet together at Wayne's new place. This solution was the opposite of what had been happening to date, where the focus had been on Wayne returning to the hostel (leading to arguments and to him "getting into trouble"). Now they proposed stepping into the community together, with Ruth visiting Wayne.

The third and fourth sessions will not be described here as they mainly focused upon staff members listening to Wayne's and Ruth's points of view, as described in the first and second sessions.

* * *

Fifth session: Ruth and Wayne invited their mother along and used the session to ask her to help them get their father to understand that they were independent and were managing well on their own and that they wanted him to treat them as adults not as children. Their mother was genuinely pleased about their progress. She was also pleased to hear that Ruth and Wayne wished to spend time together as a family. Following comments by the reflecting team, Ruth and Wayne were able to reframe their father's behaviour. They now considered that his "telling us what to do to" might be his way of showing concern: "He cares for us and wants us to do it right." They arranged to visit home when their father was there and not, as they had been doing, just visit their mother. They were also able to say to their mother how worried they were about their father's health, which had always been a taboo subject since his industrial injury and which Ruth and Wayne had only talked about in their sessions with us and not elsewhere. They decided to take a break from family therapy after session five.

Summary of sessions

Working systemically allowed Wayne and Ruth to work together on their issues, as brother and sister and as independent adults. Involving other parts of their system in this collaborative work effected change in the wider system. On the one hand, it helped care staff accept that whatever degree of independence Wayne and Ruth achieved, staff needed to take account of their relationship. In terms of affecting the wider family, the session that involved their mother facilitated Wayne's and Ruth's return to the family as independent adults in their own right and not only as children of their parents.

Reflections from members of the participating family and care system

One of the authors (who had not been involved at the time of therapy) conducted a series of consultations with Ruth, Wayne, and two care staff (who had attended some sessions) in order to gather a range of perspectives on their experience of family therapy. Ruth, Wayne, and the care staff were seen separately. Their reflections about the therapy process are presented in their own words. The quotes have been shortened, without affecting the overall meaning.

Reflections from Ruth

"It's good, I liked going. I liked talking about my anger and problems, ... Mum and Dad ..."

"I didn't feel worried ... the mirror was great. They used to record us, it was interesting. I liked it with the team. The team were asking questions to Colin. ... He wrote things down. I liked there being more people as they helped out by listening, and they were interested."

"At first I felt a bit embarrassed, and didn't know what to say. But then I asked questions, and it felt OK."

"Sometimes I took breaks if I felt restless, and got some fresh air and water."

"I still get angry and argue with my brother, but now we get on better."

"Talking with one another helped. I would tell a friend it's O.K. to go."

Reflections from Wayne

"It was OK. They were friendly people."

"Colin told us about the head mike [sic], speakers, people behind the screen—it didn't bother me."

"I felt nervous at the beginning, just sitting there and talking, camera, but it wore off after a bit. I liked seeing it recorded on video."

"Talked about family, Mum, Dad and sister. Colin wanted to know about our family, relationships, and problems."

"Everything was OK. Didn't need to change it. Could follow what was said OK. Surprised by cameras and microphones, but thought it was OK, a good surprise."

"It was good to have the chance to talk with Mum there."

"Having staff there helped at the beginning as didn't know what it would turn out like ... helped me relax ... say a few words. Staff didn't know what to expect either."

"Helped letting things out, not to bottle things up, so that people who were there could hear what we were saying."

"It would help a friend."

Reflections from care staff

Two members of care staff who supported Ruth and Wayne spoke about their experience of the sessions. They had noticed the therapy was helpful for Ruth and Wayne particularly around issues such as relationship difficulties with each other; the relationship with their father; transition from home to independent living; and authority and control. The latter referred to the relationship between Ruth, Wayne, and care-staff and to negotiating increasing autonomy. They felt that it was important for Ruth and Wayne to find a space to speak openly to each other.

* * *

The care staff's comments largely focused on their own experience of attending the sessions. Initially they felt that their role should have been supportive, simply helping Ruth and Wayne to attend, rather than directly participating in the sessions themselves. This seemed to be related to the ambiguity of their role and to ambivalent feelings about seeing themselves as part of the system. They had, at times, felt "under the spotlight", "uncomfortable", and "like a fish out of water". However, they recalled becoming aware that some of the relationship difficulties between Ruth and Wayne were due to the effects of service provision and that they themselves were part of that context.

* * *

In summary, the reflecting-team method was perceived as "strange" initially by all participants. However, the time given to explanations about the set-up supported people's adjustment. The listening skills and questions of the reflecting team, the chance to talk with the lead practitioner, and the involvement of people with whom they shared important relationships were regarded as significant elements in gaining benefit from the sessions. The service users commented that they actually liked having more people present who were interested in them.

Reflections from the Leeds FPTS

The team was consulted about their experiences of working with people with intellectual disabilities, their families, and care-systems. Although only some practitioners had been members of the team working with Ruth and Wayne, the majority had some experience of working with people with intellectual disabilities. This is not surprising given that an audit of referrals (1998–99), found that 11% of all referrals involved a person with intellectual disabilities (Houghton, 1999).

* * *

First, practitioners were asked to reflect upon their thoughts and feelings prior to using family therapy with people with intellectual disabilities. For some people, there had been a concern that the individuals' level of ability might have implications for informed consent, with regard to participating in the therapy process and fully understanding what was taking place. There had also been a concern that their ability to engage might be constrained. Some team members' only previous experience with people with intellectual disabilities had been in medical settings with people who were aggressive and self-harming. Consequently, they wondered how suitable the approach might be and whether they might find the experience too stressful. However, most team members had experience of working with the impact of chronic difficulties on people's lives. They were familiar with communication difficulties, memory problems, restricted lifestyles, and dependence upon care systems, as these factors are not unique to people with intellectual disabilities (Furlong, Young, Perlesz, McLachlan, & Reiss, 1991). They therefore concluded that these concerns related not only to clients with intellectual disabilities and that more clinical skills were transferable than they had previously recognized.

Second, practitioners reflected on their experiences of using family therapy with groups or families where a member had intellectual disabilities. There was agreement that initial concerns had not been realized and that, instead, general issues (such as finding a space to talk about difficult issues) were more salient than the intellectual disability per se. It was essential at the beginning of therapy to include carers and workers from the wider system and to address their concerns about what family therapy would involve. By including care staff and family, the team had an awareness of how people were talked about within the system, the restrictive and problem-saturated stories created around the person with intellectual disabilities, and the huge impact upon their lives and self-perceptions. The focus of the work, therefore, was often on changing the dialogue and moving away from problem-saturated stories. Like themselves, the team found that initially carers underestimated the capacity of individuals to use family therapy and were surprised by the abilities and involvement of the person with intellectual disabilities. Care staff often commented that they would take this new understanding back to the home setting.

* * *

There was some need to adapt therapeutic techniques (e.g., to write things down, slow the pace of therapy, give extra practical help with reminders for appointments and transport). However, adaptations often have to be made for other families to meet individual needs. For example, people with a head injury, those with dementia, and young children often require things to be made concrete and to have practical aids to remembering and so forth. Most importantly, working systemically with people with intellectual disabilities enabled the team to look beyond the "label" and move away from a disability discourse.

The team members considered overarching themes in therapy and whether these themes were the same or different when clients had intellectual disabilities. Universal themes that were particularly pertinent were belonging and separation; risk and protection; and the responsibilities of other family members when parents were no longer around. These themes are concerned with the values and commitments of individuals and the dynamics of relationships within the family.

Two areas of difference emerged from the discussion. First, in contrast to other groups, different workers attended the session with the person with intellectual disabilities, and so there was less consistency in sessions. Second, there was a sense that the relationship between the team and people with intellectual disabilities was more emotionally laden. For both the team and the person with intellectual disabilities, the experience of therapy can be intensely and mutually enriching. The reflecting-team approach appeared to provide people with intellectual disabilities with an empowering and novel experience of being heard. For the team, it provided a context in which we could address, in some small way, the marginalization of people's lives.

One of the main outcomes of therapy identified by the team was seeing changes in the care staff and how they understood the difficulties. One way this was evidenced was through a change in the dialogue and how the person with intellectual disabilities was spoken about. Initially language tended to be paternalistic and limiting, but gradually it became more empowering and collaborative. As sessions progressed, carers displayed a greater awareness about how their own behaviour, or that of the wider system, might be maintaining or exacerbating difficulties, and they were attempting changes in response to this. There was a shift away from scapegoating and a blaming, problem-saturated narrative to one where abilities, strengths, and resources were recognized. According to the team members we interviewed, the overall experience of working with care systems and people with intellectual disabilities had been positive and encouraging.

Conclusion

In our experience, family therapy is an approach that people with intellectual disabilities can benefit from, participate in, and feel comfortable with. Across the lifespan, irrespective of client group, the themes that emerge in therapy differ little—for example, transition, loss, protection, and fear of the future and change (Goldberg et al., 1995). Likewise, the attributes and resources that facilitate solutions—such as resilience, creativity, determination, personal development, and aspiration—are also present in the systems that include people with intellectual disabilities.

* * *

It is helpful, although not essential, to have a practitioner from the intellectual disability service within the team. This person can advise on communication difficulties and will have a familiarity with day services and other specialist provision. Although those who were not working in intellectual disability services were anxious about their ability in this area when the team first started, this soon changed. What seemed to be more important was having the ability to help clients feel safe and secure, a curiosity and willingness to struggle to understand what was being told, and an ability to adjust the process and the pace to meet individual needs. There were significant personal and professional benefits to practitioners in becoming familiar with other services and getting to know different client groups.

* * *

In the course of our experience over the last ten or so years, we have found that the techniques of systemic therapy—for example, co-construction, circular questioning, and the use of the reflecting team—are particularly relevant to people with intellectual disabilities. This client group are often accomplished in communicating their issues through metaphor and story (Sinason, 1992), which can be the building blocks of co-constructing their preferred identities (White, 1995). Circular questioning allows them to listen to and to comment on other people's perspectives on sensitive issues in a supportive rather than confrontational context. Additionally, models of systemic therapy that respect each person as the expert on their own lives resonate with people who rarely get heard and are very aware of issues of power and disempowerment (White & Epston, 1990). We believe this approach provides a more effective framework for successful therapy, as it considers the wider system within its remit—for example, individual, couple, family, and professional. Moreover, in our experience, service users are able to be involved in all of these discussions and interventions, if they so choose. To date, the people with intellectual disabilities who have attended Leeds FPTS have had mild or moderate intellectual disabilities. As a team we are interested in ways in which this approach can be made more accessible to people less able to tell their story—those with severe and profound intellectual disabilities. From the viewpoint of team development, it is of utmost importance that a lifespan team, which includes professionals with a variety of perspectives, spends time regularly discussing the concepts, theories, and techniques that they use when working as a team. This, along with discussion of areas of difference or concern, enhances team members' sense of trust when working together and facilitates the co-creation of a coherent understanding of the therapeutic processes and goals. As a result team members feel supported in their work and are more able to make use of live supervision within the session. A lifespan context is inherently diverse and intrinsically values multiple perspectives. Practitioners' specialist knowledge and expertise varies greatly from family to family. Therefore, our appreciation of our own expertise and of families' and other team members' expertise is enhanced.

Recommendations for future service development

The lifespan and inclusive nature of the team is viewed as its main asset and is something to which every member of the team is committed. This requires management understanding and support, because by its nature it is about interdisciplinary and cross-specialist working. Audit and evaluation are therefore important tasks for the team to undertake to ensure managers are aware of the value of a lifespan approach.

The term "family" therapy might be confusing and may not convey that the approach can be used with groups of people, such as service users and care teams (Quarry & Burbach, 1998; Rhodes, 2000) (see also chapter 8). Information for carers and service users should give examples of the varied ways in which the systemic approach can be offered.

In the future we would like to explore additional ways of increasing the accessibility and flexibility of the service. For example, we would like to offer consultations to staff teams to discuss how the approach could be tailored to their requirements. We are interested in ways that the reflecting team might be used to provide supervision to other teams and systemic practitioners (Fox, Tench, & Marie, 2002). We also want to develop our cultural sensitivity by making links with translators, signers, community elders, and other teams nationally and internationally.

Key learning points in setting up a lifespan service

- If you are a small service, working across the lifespan may be the most feasible and cost-effective way of delivering family therapy.
- Consider where your team would fit in with local need and other service provision and ensure that you are part of the system and are supported by it.
- Find interested people in key service areas who use systemic approaches for support, discussion, and development.
- Obtain and maintain management agreement and support for working in this way—for example, lifespan family therapy teams meet *Valuing People* (Department of Health, 2001) and *National Service Framework* (Department of Health, 1999) targets for working with carers as well as service users.

- Apply the model to yourself in working practices (e.g., training, supervision, research).
- Audit, evaluate and disseminate work to others (and be prepared to write about it).
- Involve students and trainees: as well as helping with evaluation, they have fresh perspectives to offer families and teams.
- Involve service users in the development of the service.
- Keep inspired (e.g., networking, training days, away-days).

CHAPTER FOUR

Setting up and evaluating a family therapy service in a community team for people with intellectual disabilities

Sandra Baum and Sarah Walden

Over the last few years, the clinical psychology team in Newham (an inner-city London borough) has developed a family therapy service for adults with intellectual disabilities and their families. This initiative stemmed from an increasing awareness that people with intellectual disabilities live within a complex system of carers, services, and agencies and, as such, sometimes encounter difficulties that can best be understood from a systemic perspective.

* * *

As well as an awareness of the complexity of systems within which people live, the team was also struck by an increasing number of client referrals where, upon assessment, "family issues" appeared to be prominent. These included "chronic sorrow" (Wikler, Waslow, & Hatfield, 1981); grief for the loss of a "perfect child" (Bicknell, 1983); dismay at the loss of an "ordinary life" for the family (Vetere, 1993); anxieties about "perpetual parenthood" (Todd & Shearn, 1996); and transitional issues and out-of-synchrony life-cycle events—particularly in relation to the adult with intellectual disabilities leaving home (Goldberg et al., 1995). This suggested that a systemic perspective with a focus on the system, and on interactions and relationships between

SETTING UP AND EVALUATING A FAMILY THERAPY SERVICE   65

parts of the system, might well be helpful in work with such families. Furthermore, some of the re-referrals received by the clinical psychology team indicated that this approach might be helpful. These re-referrals typically occurred after individual psychological interventions had been completed during the previous year using specific psychological models, including behavioural models (La Vigna & Donnellan, 1986); cognitive behavioural models (Stenfert Kroese, 1997); and psychodynamic models (Sinason, 1992; Beail, 1995). Many of these re-referrals focused on "family issues", which family members often felt ready to talk about, as they appeared to have had a positive experience of previous psychological interventions. This highlighted the need for an additional, alternative, psychological approach that could complement the individual work that had already been carried out with the client.

* * *

This chapter is an attempt by two of the team members to describe the process whereby a family therapy service for adults with intellectual disabilities and their families was created. We focus on the key events together with some of the obstacles and challenges that were faced on the way. Finally, we explore some ideas about how this kind of service can be evaluated in order to help us shape the service as it evolves into the future.

Setting up a systemic therapy service

Initial stages of developing the service

At the time we set up the service, the Newham clinical psychology team for people with intellectual disabilities comprised six trained clinical psychologists, each at different stages of their psychology careers—from newly qualified psychologists to a consultant clinical psychologist. At any one time the team had two trainee clinical psychologists on placement. As such, the team was a mix of individuals, predominantly white females, with multiple professional influences. These included different levels of training in systemic practice, ranging from that provided on doctorate clinical psychology training courses to introductory- and intermediate-level training courses in systemic therapy. It also included different clinical, management, and supervision experiences and, of course, multiple personal influences (such as our own experiences of being in families and our beliefs about individual and family functioning).

* * *

Traditionally, each member of the team worked individually, with all qualified staff receiving supervision from the consultant clinical psychologist, and giving supervision to trainees. Regular discussion of our practice took place, both formally, at referral and review meetings, and informally, as a result of shared offices, conversations in corridors, the need to de-brief after difficult meetings, and so forth. Such discussions enabled us to express our views about our frustrations of trying to work with people who live in complex systems and about the need for an alternative approach. As a team we had these conversations within the wider context of a district psychology and counselling service that had a history of working systemically with adults with mental health problems (Partridge, Bennett, Webster, & Ekdawi, 1995; Ekdawi, Gibbons, Bennett, & Hughes, 2000). This context and "culture" of the service supported us in considering a systemic way of working, and a systemic practitioner from the adult mental health team agreed to have initial consultations with us about the application of this approach in our speciality.

We were inspired by these initial consultations and consequently carried out an informal audit of our experiences of working systemically and of our systemic theoretical knowledge. This revealed that, as a whole, the team had had exposure to a broad base of different theoretical approaches, including structural (Minuchin, 1974), Milan (Boscolo, Cecchin, Hoffman, & Penn, 1987), post-Milan (Cecchin, Lane, & Ray, 1992), and narrative approaches (Freedman & Combs, 1996). Such a range and diversity of knowledge was a real impetus for the team—we felt that we knew something about systemic working and that it was worth sharing our knowledge, skills, and expertise to further develop as a team.

* * *

We agreed to use the format employed by our colleagues in the adult mental health service when conducting family sessions—that of a lead practitioner with a reflecting team in the room (Andersen, 1987, 1991)—as we did not have access to one-way mirrors. We were also mindful that people with intellectual disabilities were likely to have had many experiences of being observed and "judged", which in turn might raise anxieties if we were to use one-way mirrors. The approach entails the reflecting team observing the family interview and then discussing the interview among themselves, commenting on the interview in a way that both highlights the family's strengths and opens up new possibilities for problem resolution. Crucially, the family observes the discussion of the reflecting team. Following the reflection, the family and the lead practitioner resume the session and discuss any ideas that may have come from listening to the observations of the reflecting team. We also used a four-part session comprising a pre-session (30 minutes), a session with the family, which incorporates a reflecting team discussion (90 –120 minutes), and a post-session discussion (30 minutes).

* * *

From our initial discussions it quickly became apparent that it was vital for the team to have an external supervisor to guide the therapeutic work, to add to the team's ideas and knowledge base, as well as to highlight different theoretical approaches, methods, and techniques. The team accessed an external supervisor who worked with adults with mental health problems within the broader psychology and counselling service; she was a clinical psychologist and a qualified systemic practitioner, and she agreed to supervise the team for a monthly three-hour session.

There were some anxieties within the team about working in this way. For many of us it was our first experience of working therapeutically with other clinical psychologists. The idea that as practitioners we might be "found out" or "exposed as useless" was jokingly discussed in our initial conversations. This thought quickly disappeared as we realized that working in this way meant that we had the skills and knowledge of each other to draw on as a resource and support when dealing with particularly complex issues.

Referral procedure

At the time when we established the new service, the multidisciplinary community team accepted referrals after two team members had completed an "initial contact assessment". This was a generic assessment, collecting information about the demographics of the person concerned; details about the reason for referral; a description of the difficulties and needs of the person; and a recommendation regarding which discipline was the most appropriate to take the referral forward.

If, after receiving the "initial contact assessment", we considered that the persons' difficulties could best be understood within the family context rather than at an individual level, then family therapy was considered as an approach and was offered. Our impressions of how the family perceived their offspring's difficulties were an important part of this decision process—for example, if it was obvious that the families perceived all the problems as located "within their son/daughter", then a systemic approach might not work for the family. Another consideration was whether the family was "ready" for systemic work. As practitioners, we may perceive that relationship issues are key in the family, but raising these issues within the family if they are not at a stage to discuss them may cause anxiety and, consequently, an avoidance of systemic work (Vetere & Dallos, 2003). In these two instances, the most helpful approach might well be to start with some individually focused work with the person with intellectual disabilities in order to engage with the family before suggesting other work such as family therapy. However, we are always mindful that such an approach may reinforce a family's tendency to locate all problems within the intellectually disabled member, and thus we continually reflect and examine the impact of our work when faced with such dilemmas.

* * *

The main criterion used to determine whether family therapy was a useful way of addressing a referral was to ascertain whether difficulties experienced by the adult with intellectual disabilities are best understood within a family or wider context. The issues already described were helpful in this decision-making process, as were discussions within supervision. Obviously, we could only work in this way with families if they consented to family therapy. To introduce this way of working, we sent out an information sheet with the initial appointment letter. When families attended the initial appointment (either in their home or at our base), we expanded on the idea further and gained their verbal consent to work in this way.

In the early days, we decided to work primarily with families where English was the first language because we considered that working systemically with interpreters would initially be too much of a challenge for us. Raval (1996, 2003) outlines some of the issues that practitioners can face when working systemically with interpreters. The therapy can be experienced by the practitioners as being slower and less effective, and there can be difficulties for the interpreter in translating directly, with semantic changes needing to be made in order for the interpreter to make sense to the family. Raval (1996) also states that "techniques such as circular questioning, enactment, use of a reflecting team or intensification may be more difficult to use with an interpreter" (p. 37). As we considered ourselves novices in these techniques, we decided to proceed wearily. We have subsequently developed our confidence and now find working with interpreters to be less of a challenge. Indeed, we have found that it often gives the intellectually disabled member the chance to hear the dialogue and reflections twice and thus may increase the possibility of comprehension.

Role of lead practitioner

During the team's preliminary discussions, it was agreed that the lead practitioner and reflecting team would have specific roles. The lead practitioner was to have organizational responsibility for the session (in terms of booking the therapy space) and any contact with the family outside of the session (e.g., writing and sending appointment letters, making any necessary telephone calls, etc.). Within the session the lead practitioner was to have responsibility for informing the family about the format, the role of the reflecting team, and issues of confidentiality, as well as facilitating and leading the conversation. The lead practitioner would also coordinate the completion of the session notes, including the pre-session discussion, content of the session, and post-session discussion.

Role of reflecting team

The reflecting team's tasks included taking part in the pre-session discussion with the lead practitioner about the family and their presenting problem, as well as developing initial hypotheses to guide the lead practitioner's questions during the session. The reflecting team also took notes during the session. Any questions that the reflecting team had for the family were communicated through the lead practitioner (i.e., the reflecting-team member asked the lead practitioner to ask the family a specific question). The reflecting team was also vital during the post-session discussion to reflect on the session and further develop any hypotheses that had arisen.

The main role of the reflecting team, however, was to reflect on the session at an appropriate stage as it unfolded, sometimes with the lead practitioner, sometimes without, depending on the number of reflecting-team members and the content of the session. Andersen (1987, 1991) suggests some parameters for reflecting teams. Reflections should include a small number of team members (no more than three); be speculative; be given in the style of the family's normal speech; be relevant to the preceding conversation; and not differ too much from the family's current views. He classifies three types of reflection: those commenting on the picture of the problem situation; the ways in which family members have constructed their picture of the problem; and the ways in which family members might construct new pictures of the problem. An example of a meaningful reflection for one family was when the issue of a short break was being discussed for the 27-year-old daughter with severe intellectual disabilities of elderly parents. The parents had constructed a picture that sending their daughter away for a short break would be seen as them failing to care for her within the family home. One reflecting-team member speculatively raised the idea that short breaks could be very positive for people with intellectual disabilities, as it enabled them to have different experiences, make new friends, and so on. Once the session resumed, the family discussed this extensively with the lead practitioner as being something that they had not considered, and this subsequently led them to try this idea out.

Organizing sessions with families

Two sessions with different families were initially timetabled into a weekly slot of four hours. Four sub-teams were created, each with a lead practitioner and at least two reflecting-team members. However, due to the needs of the families and of the team members, flexibility became a key issue, and families were seen on a monthly basis but at a time that was mutually convenient for the families and the sub-teams.

Site for therapy

Families were seen either at our office premises, which had to provide a therapeutic space big enough to encompass the family, the lead practitioner, and the reflecting team or, alternatively, in their home. The latter arrangement was common for families where there were mobility problems, or where the parents' advancing age and associated health problems meant it was not feasible for them to travel.

Supervision

The importance of supervision was referred to earlier in the chapter. Supervision included discussion of possible referrals to the service and whether this way of working would be useful for certain families or particular presenting problems. A large part of the time was spent reflecting on sessions with families, formulating hypotheses and questions for use in further sessions, as well as developing the team members' skills as practitioners by considering what might have been done differently within sessions. The supervision process was, hopefully, a mutually rewarding experience, highlighting for our supervisor and us some of the similarities that people with intellectual disabilities and adults with mental health problems experience in the context of their families and wider systems.

Obstacles and challenges

After some months of operating this service, the team members took some time to reflect on their experiences, particularly the obstacles and challenges. This focused, as discussed in what follows, on the site for therapy; including the person with intellectual disabilities; the agenda for change; and involving members of the wider system.

Site for therapy

As highlighted earlier, the therapeutic work sometimes took place in people's homes. While such an arrangement can be advantageous in terms of having access to a broader view of people's circumstances, and potentially a greater degree of familiarity and intimacy with families (Snyder & McCollum, 1999), it can also present challenges to the usual boundaries inherent in working in a clinical setting. There can be a shift in power as a result of being on the client's "home turf", with strong cultural values prevailing about how to behave as "a visitor". The team was faced with an ongoing challenge of how to maintain essential therapeutic boundaries while being respectful of the clients' space. Interruptions to sessions in terms of other visitors and telephone calls were common, as was the issue of "who's in charge of the physical space" (Snyder & McCollum, 1999) in relation to, for example, the seating arrangements. One family rearranged the furniture between every session, providing the team members with the problem on an ongoing basis of where to sit and how to ensure that every member of the family could take part in the session.

* * *

Confidentiality can also be compromised when working in people's homes. Visitors who were in the home with the permission of the family—for example, neighbours or tradespeople—presented challenges to the (therapeutic) notion of confidentiality. We attempted to overcome such issues by making explicit agreements or contracts with families prior to beginning sessions. These referred to boundaries and to the parameters that needed to be adhered to and, in general, aimed to ensure that the sessions ran smoothly and were of maximum use to the families. However, throughout the work such agreements needed to be referred to regularly with the families.

Including the person with intellectual disabilities

Including the person with intellectual disabilities in systemic work can be a challenge. Fidell (2000) argues that it would be discriminatory not to include clients in sessions, but care must be taken to avoid their presence being "tokenistic". We spent considerable time in pre-sessions and supervision thinking of the different ways that this might be achieved, and some of our conclusions are as follows.

It is vital to be aware of the language being used in sessions and to make attempts to tailor it to the client's comprehension and communication abilities. Circular questioning can be complex to understand, as it requires people to be able to step outside of a relationship and become an observer. Our work, however, indicated that some clients were able to respond to certain types of circular questions—for example, "Who is most worried in the family?" Fidell (1996) also describes certain techniques and tools that can be used to include people with intellectual disabilities in systemic sessions, citing drawings, symbols, role play, pictorial ladders to help with ranking, and so on. (These ideas are further developed in chapters five and ten.)

We also used the reflecting team to focus on the individual's perspectives during sessions. This was particularly useful for observing the client and monitoring if he or she was losing interest and so forth. Our experience indicated that there were clear advantages to having clients present within the session, as they were more likely to give spontaneous accounts of what was happening within the family. There was also an advantage for us as practitioners in observing how the family interacted as a system, focusing on its nonverbal communication as much as its verbal communication. For example, the parents of a 21-year-old man with mild intellectual disabilities, who complained that their son was immature and not "growing up", took their son's cap off and tidied his hair on a number of occasions during the sessions, and he normally sat on the floor at their feet.

* * *

One possible drawback of including people with intellectual disabilities occurs when the issue of "blame" is prominent and where a family member may thus be scapegoated during the sessions. In such situations, the parents and/or person with intellectual disabilities can be seen separately on the first few occasions, with a view to a family meeting taking place in due course (Roy-Chowdhury, 1992; Fidell, 2000). We adopted this approach with one family where the parents had strong views about the behaviour of the eldest daughter with mild intellectual disabilities (they had two daughters with intellectual disabilities). As a therapy team, we sometimes felt uncomfortable about the way the eldest daughter's behaviour was spoken about in front of her, and we felt that it was difficult for her to express her views in the sessions. We consequently arranged a session with just this daughter and her sister, who was moderately intellectually disabled, with the specific aim of engaging with them and attempting to understand their viewpoint.

Agenda for change

As already described, families did not initially request family therapy. This was perhaps due to them not knowing that this was an option for thinking about their concerns. The "need" for these meetings was always identified by the clinical psychologist. As with any psychological intervention, it is important to ensure that the agenda for change is shared. Difficulties arose when the parents' agenda for change was widely different from that of the practitioner—for example, when they wanted their offspring to be "fixed" or "cured" as a result of attending sessions. During the initial session with one family, the mother asked us whether these meetings would make her son "normal" so that he would be able to go to university like his brother. Once it was explained that we could not help them achieve such a goal, the family did not return.

In order to make the agenda for change explicit, we have been finding it extremely useful to negotiate the goals of therapy within the first few sessions. Clear goals are useful in monitoring change and in helping families and practitioners decide when therapy should come to an end. The process of negotiation is discussed in more detail in the next section.

Involving members of the wider system

People with intellectual disabilities are often part of larger networks and systems, and consequently it is important to be mindful of who else apart from the immediate family they may see as important. Our experience indicated that at times it was useful to include paid carers who also knew clients well and who could provide another perspective on the person's and family's difficulties. We have learnt that if people from the wider system are invited to the sessions, it is crucial to ensure that all parties are in agreement with this and that issues of confidentiality are made explicit.

Evaluating our work

Evaluating systemic therapy presents numerous challenges to the practitioner. The entire family may be seen and may benefit, yet there may be no adequate way of capturing how change has been accomplished. Ideally, an evaluation should provide information on symptom improvement in the identified person (first-order change) and how family relationships are organized or structured (second-order change) (Sprenkle & Moon, 1996). Assessing change in families is difficult, as most measures cannot tap subtle shifts in perceptions and attitudes that may be brought about by systemic therapy. It appears easier to measure change in individuals than in dyads or families, and therefore first-order change remains the most widely used and reliable criterion. (See Sprenkle & Moon, 1996, for further discussion of these issues.)

* * *

Evaluation measures in general must take into account the complexity of psychological interventions and therefore should not reduce clients' responses to a number, as this does not reflect the complexity of their problems. They must be able to be implemented in daily practice but can be either routine, situation-specific, periodic, or in-depth (Berger, 1996). It is preferable for the views of the person with intellectual disabilities to be sought, even though this can present a challenge to practitioners due to potential comprehension and communication difficulties (Booth & Booth, 1996). The ethics that underpin much of the practice in public funded services means that the process of how we measure our interventions is vital, in order to ensure that we are not using our power as practitioners in an overintrusive way. In view of this, it is important not to give families too many measures and for the measures to be relevant and meaningful.

Evaluation measures used

Due to the lack of suitable measures, we decided to design our own outcome tools in order to pilot an evaluation of our service, collecting data at two points in the therapeutic process—the first and last sessions. In the initial session with the family, we asked specific questions to clarify each family member's view of the problem as well as their goals for change. We also attempted to clarify the lead practitioner's and the reflecting team's perspective on the problem with the family present.

In the last session (whenever therapy had a planned ending), we focused on finding out family members' views of the therapeutic intervention—for example, whether their goals for change had been achieved, whether they had noticed any changes in their relationships and communication or any symptom reduction—as well as their views about the most and least useful aspects of the therapy. In addition, we collected routine information to provide a summary of the socio-demographic data and details of intervention of all families seen, including the number of sessions; cancellations; duration of intervention; major themes emerging in therapy; as well as the models of intervention used.

Socio-demographic data

Table 4.1 shows that nine families were seen during the evaluation pilot. In all of these, an identified person with intellectual disabilities was named, of whom six were men and four were women (two of the latter were from the same family). Three families were seen at home due to the parents' ill health, and one family was seen with an interpreter. Six of the families were seen at our office base.

Presenting problems

Information about the presenting problems was obtained from the evaluation tool completed after the first session. In three of the families, the adult with intellectual disabilities was engaging in outwardly directed behaviours such as hitting and breaking objects. In two of the families, the person with intellectual disability was verbally abusive towards others and was considered immature by their parents. In two of the families, bereavement and loss were the main reasons for referral. For two families, there were concerns regarding where the intellectually disabled person would live in the future.

Duration of work with families

Table 4.1 also shows that of the six families who completed therapy, one family was seen for nine sessions over 17 months, while the other families were seen for nine sessions over 15 months, six sessions over 11 months, seven sessions over 12 months, eight sessions over 12 months and three sessions over 5 months. Of the families who stopped attending (no reason given), two families attended one session only and one family attended two sessions.

Table 4.1. The socio-demographic data of the nine families seen by the family therapy team and duration of intervention

Family	Age of I.D. person	Gender and position in family	Degree of I.D.	Ethnic origin and religion (if known)	No. of sessions / months in therapy	No. of DNA's	Specialist resources/ equipment
1.	20	male, oldest of two	moderate	Iranian	1 / 1 month uc.c	1	interpreter
2.	23	male, only son	mild	white British	7 / 12 months c.c	2	home visits due to father's ill-health
3.	27	female, third child	severe	white British	3 / 5 months c.c	0	home visits due to father's ill-health
4.	23	male, youngest of two	mild	white British	9 / 15 months (father died after 5 sessions) c.c	3	home visits due to father's ill-health
5.	17	female, oldest of four	mild–moderate	white British	1 / 1 month uc.c	1	N/A
6.	44	male twin (they are oldest of six children)	mild–moderate	white British	2 / 7 months uc.c	3	N/A
7.	22 19	female, oldest; female, youngest	mild; moderate–severe	Pakistani Muslim	9 / 17 months c.c	4	N/A
8.	22	male, oldest of three children	mild	Indian–Punjabi Hindu	6 / 11 months c.c	1	N/A
9.	39	male, youngest of four children	mild	white British	8 / 12 months c.c	1	N/A

Key: I.D. = intellectual disabilities; DNA = did not attend; O.T. = occupational therapist; c.c = completed family therapy sessions. Case closed, uc.c = uncompleted family therapy sessions; family did not attend further sessions.

Themes and models of working

For five of the families, the life-cycle transition from childhood to adulthood was relevant. Other pertinent themes were that three of the parents were suffering from life-threatening illnesses, with one father dying during the course of therapy. Bereavement and loss were also significant themes for some of the families, with the concept of "chronic sorrow" (Wikler, Waslow, & Hatfield, 1981) being relevant for five families. Other themes were issues of triangulation or scapegoating (Roy-Chowdhury, 1992) for three families; marital difficulties for two families; sibling relationships for three families; fear of violence for two families; and parents feeling "captive" or "captivated" (Todd & Shearn, 1996) in three families. Information given by the systemic therapy team in relation to services available was relevant for two families. The therapeutic models employed by the team were predominantly derived from Milan systemic therapy (Boscolo et al., 1987) and post-Milan therapy (Cecchin, Lane, & Ray, 1992).

Outcomes

Information about outcome was obtained from the evaluation tool completed during and after the final session. Out of the nine families seen during the pilot stage, for the six families who completed therapy, the goals identified were achieved. Three families only attended one or two sessions and did not return for further appointments.

From the data collected, it appears that goals identified in the first session were achieved by all of those families who engaged with the process and completed therapy. Some families reported symptom reduction in outwardly directed behaviour by the adults with intellectual disabilities and changes in family structure in some families. For example, in the first session, one family when asked about what their goals for change were responded:

Mother: "I want to be able to cope with my daughter's behaviour. I don't know how things could be different."

Father: "She [daughter] is very difficult in the mornings, I want things to be better."

Daughter with intellectual disabilities [no response].

* * *

In the final session, the same family commented:

> *Mother:* "Things are better. We spend more time as a couple. We have less problems in dealing with our daughter's behaviour."
>
> *Father:* "We don't argue as much. She [*daughter*] is much better."
>
> *Daughter with intellectual disabilities* [*gives the "thumbs-up" sign, as not able to communicate verbally*].

* * *

The data shows that the majority of families who engaged in therapy were seen for between six and nine sessions over 12 to 17 months. This is similar to Goldberg et al.'s (1995) observation that "The pace of therapy is often slow. The sessions themselves can appear slowed down, and the therapeutic process may be extended over many months" (p. 278). Also there are often difficulties in negotiating endings with families with an intellectually disabled member. Intellectual disability is a life-long condition, and although the therapy may have improved certain aspects of the family's situation, many issues will be unresolved due to the disability remaining (Goldberg et al., 1995; Fidell, 2000).

* * *

The team was most likely to see clients who were in their twenties. All of the nine families were in a time of transition due either to the ill health or death of a parent or to the transition between childhood to adulthood. The literature highlights that transitions can upset the homeostasis of the family because they often demand a change in how the family interacts and upsets its behaviour patterns. A family member may become "symptomatic" if the family cannot adapt to or negotiate the new transition (Carter & McGoldrick, 1989). In eight of the families, the adult with disabilities was presented as having "difficult" behaviour during such a period. (See also Jennifer Clegg and Susan King's discussion on supporting people in transition, in chapter seven.)

Critique of the evaluation pilot

The preceding sections have outlined how the service was set up, how it operated in its early years, and how we attempted to evaluate it. The service is still ongoing, and we are continuing to look at ways of assessing whether the service we provide is effective. We are developing our practice in an area that is traditionally difficult to evaluate (Sprenkle & Moon, 1996), with a client group that has hitherto not been included in this kind of approach. This is pioneering work and is still in progress. We have so far had encouraging feedback from the families we have worked with, which will enable us to continue to refine our methods of evaluation.

The method we used in the pilot project focused primarily on goals identified at the beginning of therapy and the achievement of these at the end of therapy. It did not focus on individual sessions or the process of therapy. Clearly this needs to be progressed. We presently record all the sessions via written notes completed during the session. However, video equipment has now been installed in the therapy room, which could allow us to analyse the process of each session in greater detail. One way of doing this might be by looking for communication patterns, emotions, and interventions in each session or by selecting an important event in the therapy to transcribe and analyse, using, for example, comprehensive process analysis (Elliot, 1989), which can attempt to assess the effective aspects of interventions.

We are considering using standardized assessment instruments that have been developed to measure change and that have been used in general systemic therapy settings (see contributions in Carr, 2000b). These instruments are designed to evaluate family strengths and needs and to help monitor the progress of the work. They can be used for observational or self-report ratings. The Beavers Interactional Scales (Beavers & Hampson, 1990) could be used as an assessment tool: this is designed for practitioners to rate the family's competence and style after an episode of family interaction is observed and also involves families in completing self–report questionnaires. It is evidently a well-documented, reliable, and valid tool (for a summary, see Beavers & Hampson, 2000) and hopefully could prove useful.

We are also keen to develop self-report measures for adults with intellectual disabilities and other members of the family, and we would like to use measures of change based on drawings, symbols, and visual aids (see Fidell, 1996) to fully include the adult with intellectual disabilities in the process. This presents us with further challenges about how we actively engage people with intellectual disabilities in the process of evaluation.

One of our trainee psychologists has recently completed her doctoral dissertation on asking people with intellectual disabilities and their families (from five districts including Newham) about the experience of family therapy and whether they found it useful or not, and the results of this will hopefully inform the development of our service too (see Arkless, 2005).

Conclusions of the evaluation

Methods of evaluating the impact of systemic therapy for adults with intellectual disabilities and their families are still in the early stage of development. Clearly one of the main challenges is how we attempt to do this. There is much for us to learn about our techniques, how we include the person with intellectual disabilities, what kind of approach is most beneficial for which family, and which tools can be easily administered in a busy health-service setting. Chase and Holmes (1990) warn clinicians attempting to evaluate systemic therapy that "they will meet criticism of their methods; if not, they may be accused of cowardice" (p. 239). We have certainly striven to meet this challenge and so far have had some encouraging results.

Conclusions

This chapter describes the journey we took in setting up a systemic therapy service in a community team for people with intellectual disabilities. We have described the process we went through in setting up the service and the obstacles and challenges we faced on the way, as well as our attempts to evaluate the service.

* * *

Writing this chapter has given us the opportunity to reflect on the progress that we have made on our journey in relation to the skills we have learnt, the families we have worked with, and some of the goals that the families have achieved. Using a systemic approach with this client group has been incredibly useful, liberating, challenging, satisfying, and at times nerve-wracking! Not only has it given us an additional psychological approach to offer clients and their carers, but it has also equipped us with an alternative way of thinking about the referrals we receive and the work we do. We still have some way to go on our journey in terms of further developing our systemic skills, particularly in working with interpreters, in striving to include people with intellectual disabilities in systemic work, and, of course, in continuing to evaluate our efforts.

* * *

Perhaps the most important aspect to have come out of this journey is that we are moving further away from what Fredman (2001) describes as "the conversation of impossibility" (p. 5) that surrounds systemic work—that is, the idea that in order to be working systemically, one needs to be a fully trained and qualified family practitioners, using one-way screens, with families who all attend every session and are verbal, articulate, and intelligent. Our experience indicates that working systemically is much more about being interested, enthusiastic, respectful, willing to learn, and having appropriate guidance and systemic supervision.

How to get started with developing a systemic therapy service

- Make contact with colleagues within your context who are interested in working systemically.
- "Audit" your systemic knowledge, experience, and interest—you may be pleasantly surprised by what you find!
- Access systemic supervision—there may be someone within your wider service setting, or professional groups, who is willing to supervise you or at least have initial conversations with you about your ideas.
- Start small—identify one or two examples of work where a systemic approach may be appropriate, to allow you to develop your confidence.
- Keep managers informed about what you are doing—they may be able to let you know if there are any monies available for supervision costs, training, and so forth.
- Evaluate your work—it shows managers that working systemically is worthwhile.

CHAPTER FIVE

Engaging people with intellectual disabilities in systemic therapy

Denise Cardone and Amanda Hilton

This chapter describes how we have engaged people with intellectual disabilities in a systemic therapeutic process. We discuss here our work context and the social constructionist theory that informs our practice, using examples from our practice throughout. To more fully illustrate our approach and practice, the chapter concludes with a detailed example of our work with someone with significant intellectual and communication disabilities.

Our context

Our stories begin separately. Initially we worked as clinical psychologists with people with intellectual disabilities in two different National Health Service organizations. Independently, we had started to question traditional ways of working—the theories and models that were informing the ways we both worked as clinical psychologists. Many models of psychology, in common with the models that shape the practices of other disciplines, adopt an approach that sees the individual in isolation from the relationships and contexts that, in our view, have a powerful effect on peoples' lives and presentations. These bias an individual approach of assessment and diagnosis (i.e., to discover and label a truth) and treatment (according to this truth) of an individual or group. We became increasingly interested in what systemic models had to offer to our understanding and facilitation of change within complex systems and relationships. After meeting, sharing our thoughts, and proposing the idea of working together as a small systemic team, we wondered for some time how we might achieve this, considering the geographical and organizational barriers we faced. However, our conversations continued, and our excitement, enthusiasm, interest, and curiosity about the helpfulness of drawing on systemic ideas grew. Soon our talks became more dominated by "Why (ever) not?" and then this became "We will!" "We will" has now become "We are". We were able to empower ourselves to take our first tentative steps across the barriers of change towards organizing ourselves in a new and different way of working within the same system and organization. We created a clinic-based systemic service for children and adults with intellectual disabilities and their significant others. The process we went through in the creation of our service is one that we hoped would be mirrored in our conversations with clients. We hoped to facilitate conversations that they might find useful in co-creating a different way of looking at where they are, where they might like to be, and how they might begin to take their first steps through "barriers" to find a different way of being with each other. Initially, we found starting a systemic therapeutic service a confusing task as there are many systemic models and little in the literature to indicate which of these might be most useful in working with people with intellectual disabilities. The next two sections outline our approach and practice.

Approach

The systemic theories to which we were attracted were informed by social constructionism. Social constructionism proposes that the development of knowledge is a social phenomenon, with our beliefs about the world being social inventions having evolved in the context of verbal and nonverbal communication with others. "Truth" is not discovered but constructed by communities of people in conversation (Hoffman, 1993; Carr, 2000a). For example, ideas, truths, self-identities, and so forth are the products of human relationships. This is a bias towards multiple authorships as opposed to individual authorships: everything is authored in a community of persons and relationships (Anderson, 1995). The ideas that inform social constructionism are endorsed by many of the "second-order" family therapists (explained below), including the Milan systemic therapists, Tom Andersen's reflecting-team group, and Harry Goolishian, Harlene Anderson, Michael White, and David Epston (Andersen, 1987; White & Epston, 1990; Campbell, Draper, & Crutchley, 1991; Anderson & Goolishian, 1992; Anderson, 1995). Lynn Hoffman (1985, 1993) describes second-order practice as including "considering the therapist's context as part of the observing system; working towards collaborative, rather than a hierarchical structure; setting a context for change rather than specifying a direction for change; guarding against too much instrumentality; making a circular assessment of the problem; and, holding a non-pejorative, non-judgemental view" (quoted in Perlesz, Young, Paterson, & Bridge, 1994, p. 117).

* * *

In reviewing the literature on working systemically with people with intellectual disabilities, we found few articles that specifically linked social constructionist approaches to therapeutic practice. Just two articles make explicit reference to the social-constructionist-informed theories and second-order practices that we use in our own work (Goldberg et al.,1995; Fidell, 2000). Our chapter further develops Fidell's (2000) ideas by drawing on a broader range of methods and techniques, with detailed examples from practice to show additional ways of engaging people with intellectual disabilities in systemic therapy.

Practice

Working collaboratively is at the heart of many of the principles that guide policies in the intellectual disabilities field, such as inclusion, empowerment, engagement, and person-centred practice (*Valuing People*: Department of Health, 2001). Working collaboratively in a non-judgemental way is achieved not from a position as the "outside expert", but from an acknowledgement of the subjectivity of each and every point of view. This position has become known as the "not-knowing position" (Anderson, 1995) or a "non-expert" model, which makes use of the different types of expertise (local expertise) that the client and therapist bring to a session (Fredman, 1997). Instead of one person "knowing best", local expertise can be used to work on the problem together. Professional knowledge is not privileged. Ideas based on professional assumptions are introduced in a tentative way, as possibilities among many others.

* * *

As is usual in systemic practice, we invite everybody to have a say in co-creating the conversation. However, we have noticed that we give the person with intellectual disabilities *more* opportunities and time to voice his or her view in relation to the others present, resulting in a slower therapeutic process. This, as Fidell (2000) also argues, is because, "They may not be used to having a voice, particularly in the presence of their carers" (p. 313). Thus, persons with intellectual disabilities need to have time to consider their position on the issues, to express their position, and to be heard by others. We believe that the systemic session creates a forum in which people's voices can be heard in a different way and where their stories can be witnessed and acknowledged. A systemic session can contribute towards giving different weight to the views of a person with intellectual disabilities. When a context is established where things are potentially *heard* differently, this may in turn create opportunity for different forms of actions and interactions.

By way of illustration we would like to share a brief transcript of a conversation from a session with the Browning family. This involves Pete, an adult with intellectual disabilities, and Denise, the lead practitioner. Also present in the session were Pete's father (Jack), his mother (Sue), and the reflecting team (Amanda).

Pete: "I'm just going to say it . . . [*pause*] . . . he's a cock-up person, I'm sorry."

Denise: "Who is?"

Pete: "My dad."

Denise: "In what way?"

[*Silence. 10-second pause*]

Pete: "So many things [*pause*]. Sometimes I try to be myself [*10-second pause and cough*]. Sometimes . . . it's very hard to explain [*stumbles over word*], actually [*5-second pause and cough*]. I wouldn't be in this condition [*says word three times and sentence twice until he pronounces it to his satisfaction*]. Sometimes I have trouble with words."

Denise: "What do you mean by condition?"

Pete [*red in the face—looks angry*]: "I'm sorry . . ."

Denise [*notices how he looks and relates this back to the beginning of the conversation*]: I have noticed you have become red in the face. I wonder if you are angry with your dad—is that right?"

Pete: "Yes, a bit."

Denise: "Do you want to talk about that now, or would you rather not?"

Pete [*4-second pause*]: "I'm sorry, so sorry . . . 10, about 10 years ago . . . it started . . ." [*His voice drifts off and he chooses to say no more at this time—we take a pause in the session.*]

This extract demonstrates facilitating a voice for the person with intellectual disabilities by working at a pace that is sensitive to the "client" (e.g., sitting with silences and pausing with Pete while he thinks about what has been said or perhaps what he might choose to say or not say next). It also demonstrates the importance of using and staying close to the client's language (Andersen, 1992; Hoffman, 1993). Pete speaks in short, uncomplicated sentences and uses words that may have multiple meanings. There are many possibilities for understanding his words "cock-up" and "condition". Denise resists the temptation to find meaning according to her own ideas and biases; instead, she waits for Pete to give them his own meanings in his own time.

* * *

Another way we have found helpful in facilitating collaborative practice is to offer sessions in a "novel space". This is a place to meet that is unfamiliar to the family. This seems to create a new context where everyone potentially can start to reflect on patterns in their relationships. Mary, a woman with intellectual disabilities, said: "I need to get my mind unmuddled before I can talk . . . I can't think at home . . . I'm too busy . . . with the cats." Tom Andersen (1992) argues that "Those who do not know what to do, need something different", though he goes on to caution that "this something should not be too different" (p. 59). We apply Andersen's advice not only to *where* we talk, but also to *what* we talk with families about and to *how* we talk.

The use of teams

In order to create a context for collaboration, we have used a team in different ways to facilitate the process of reflexivity and to engage the person with intellectual disabilities in a meaningful way. When we work systemically with clients and families, we like to work with a team. One of the advantages of working with a team is that between us we can come up with more ideas. We believe we can be more helpful to people who consult with us when there is more than one person present. We draw on Tom Andersen's (1987) use of the reflecting-team method (for a full description, see chapter four). When working with people with intellectual disabilities we have found it important for the team to share only a limited number of ideas in each reflection (a maximum of three). We think this may be because the idea of being asked to reflect upon a conversation is new to most people with intellectual disabilities, and thus they may need more time to consider their position in relation to the ideas they have heard. When asking the family and lead practitioner to reflect upon the teams' reflection, we found it useful to ask the person with intellectual disabilities for his or her ideas first. This is because when we ask other family members first, they often make new connections to what they have heard, and it can therefore be hard for people with intellectual disabilities to follow the evolving process. In other words, the pace can easily become too fast.

* * *

Another way we have found of facilitating a "fit" of the pace of reflection between the team and the person with intellectual disabilities is for the team to present one succinct idea to each person in turn. Like other practitioners, we use this method when we feel that "the use of a reflecting team would risk confusing them by presenting a multiplicity of opinions, rather than a clear message which is our aim" (Fidell, 2000, p. 315). A final method for slowing down the reflecting process is to use "live consultation" (Kingston & Smith, 1985). A team of two sit in the room with the family group. One team member ("the lead practitioner") talks with the family while the other ("the consultant") listens, observes, and addresses the lead practitioner during the session with new ideas, specific questions, or more lengthy conversation to explore an idea with the lead practitioner that the family can listen to. Furthermore, the consultant often pays attention to the particular language, pace, and ideas of the person with intellectual disabilities.

This enables people with intellectual disabilities to be actively involved in the co-creation of new ideas, as they "lead" the process and pace of generating ideas.

* * *

The following example seeks to highlight some of the ideas in the previous two sections—particularly the idea of taking a non-expert view and co-creating a conversation (i.e., giving people time to consider their position on issues, express their opinion, and be heard by others) and establishing a context in which things are potentially heard differently. Richard and Sarah, both of whom had intellectual disabilities, expressed a wish to get married. The referral letter from the social worker stated that Richard's mother, Sarah's mother, and Richard's keyworker all had widely different views about the marriage which they had not shared with each other, nor with Richard or Sarah. Both Sarah's mother and Richard's keyworker wanted a psychologist's "expert opinion" about whether the couple were both capable of consenting to marriage. We invited Richard, Sarah, both their mothers, and the keyworker to meet with us. At this meeting everyone shared their views with each other for the first time. This sharing in itself made a difference: the mothers and the keyworker were able to hear Richard and Sarah's views about their relationship. Thus, they no longer felt they needed an "expert opinion" on this relationship and were able to continue to talk with each other outside the session about how they could support Richard and Sarah as a couple.

Having highlighted some general methods that we use for engaging people with intellectual disabilities in a collaborative systemic process, we now consider some more specific techniques in the form of genograms, circular questions, and the use of metaphor.

Genograms

Genograms are part of the more general process of family assessment and involve mapping family structure, recording family information, and delineating family relationships. We have found genograms to be useful when engaging with people with intellectual disabilities in systemic work. The usefulness of employing both visual and verbal modalities is well established in working with people with intellectual disabilities. Professionals have routinely used visual cues including symbols, drawings, photographs, objects, and so forth to facilitate understanding and to enhance engagement. In addition, we have found genograms to be a useful visual representation for talking about relationships and creating new ideas about relationships with people with intellectual disabilities. When creating genograms, it can often be the person with intellectual disabilities who has ideas about whom to include in the genogram, and who often has a wealth of information about who is in their family and how they are related. While people with intellectual disabilities may or may not have contact with their families, they are frequently connected with wide networks of professionals and carers. We have found that, as people tell us about the meaningful relationships in their lives, more often than not it evolves into a relationship map that includes various professionals and community networks. We have noticed that anchoring our conversations in a relationship map, co-created with the person with intellectual disabilities, enhances engagement in this process. Genograms and relationship maps can also be used to initiate discussions about "relationship to help" (Reder & Fredman, 1996). This term refers to the fact that most people who come to see us will already have had years of contact with services and a variety of professionals. We (the "clients" and the "professionals") will be bringing to the current context our beliefs about the helping process, which can significantly influence the outcome of referral and treatment (Reder & Fredman, 1996).

As we show in the next section, we may also use a genogram or relationship map as a concrete visual basis for circular questioning of relationship differences.

Circular questioning

Circular questions concern differences about people in their relationships, behaviours, speech, emotions, cognitions, intentions, events, or futures (Tomm, 1988). We have found adaptations of circular-questioning techniques for children useful in our work with people with intellectual disabilities, since the suggested contextual aides (e.g., pictures, role-play, video) address similar issues of conceptual, perceptual, and cognitive difference (Benson, Schindler-Zimmerman, & Martin, 1991).

* * *

It has been our experience that *hypothetical* circular questions of difference (i.e., questions of the "what if . . . ?" type) need to be anchored in context (i.e., person, place, and time) in order to be meaningful, since abstractions can often be difficult for people with intellectual disabilities. For example, we asked one of our clients, Christopher, "If you could be anyone in the world, *who* would you be?" We received the answer, after some thought, "My brother." We were then able to go on and explore the meaning of this. Another situation concerns linking questions to specific situations. For example, we asked one family: "If the *morning routine* could be different, how would you like it to be?" The family embarked on a lengthy conversation about what everyone would like to be different and how they could help each other to achieve this. We have also found that some people are able to say what they might wish for in the future, particularly if it is linked to a concrete event. For example, June, an adult with intellectual disabilities, her mother, Susan, her father, Graham, and her keyworker, Jimmy, attended a session with Amanda (lead practitioner). The referral letter from the social worker stated that June's keyworker, Jimmy, believed that June wanted to move from her parental home, her parents did not want her to, and arguments ensued, with June saying nothing. This led her parents to say that June did not have a view and that they knew what was best for their daughter. During the first session Amanda asked June, "If you had a magic wand and you could make things how you wanted *on your birthday*, how would that be?" June's answer was, ". . . lots of presents . . . a big cake . . . candles . . . happy . . . all happy . . . Mum, Dad, Kate, Jimmy [*staff*], Francis [*friend*] . . . party . . . garden . . . Greenfield's [*proposed new home*] . . . friends . . . lots of cards. . . ." After tearfully expressing their distress, June's parents were now able to hear that she did, after all, have her own ideas about her future.

* * *

Circular questions can also be used to explore differences in perception of magnitude between people about a given issue or event. Various pictorial representations can be used to give a description of the "size" or "scale" of the issue or concern. These include analogue scales ranging from "not at all" to a state of "maximum severity". Various emotions can be represented using symbols, photographs, or line drawings of faces. Pictures of thermometers can represent degree of "hotness" of an emotion or cognition. And, finally, there are methods unique to what clients bring, such as the clients physically demonstrating with their arms and hands how much or how little they think something effects them (Cummins, 1991; Dagnan & Ruddick, 1995; Lindsay, Neilson, &

Lawrence, 1997). In our experience, people with intellectual disabilities are able to use these methods in systemic work to converse about the news of difference between their perception and that of others. However, *ranking* seems to be a less useful method for highlighting degree differences. Questions such as, "Who is most upset when A angrily shouts at B? Who is upset next?" generally seem too complex for people with intellectual disabilities to understand. Perhaps this is because there are too many key words (ideas) per sentence. Consequently, we have adapted ranking questions for people with intellectual disabilities by asking each individual person, "On a scale from one to three, where would you be?" We then compare each person's self-rating, thus forming a ranking system.

Using circular questions to elicit the ideas and opinions of someone who is not present can be a powerful way of introducing multiple perspectives. If questions are simplified and repeated, they can be accessible—for example, "If Daisy were here now, what *might* she say?" and, "If Daisy were here now and heard you talking to Lily, what *might* she say?" This perhaps challenges some prevalent assumptions that people with intellectual disabilities are not able to think about another's point of view. In our experience, the majority of people that we have seen do seem able to hold the idea of someone absent having a point of view. We have used this successfully with several families, particularly when one member of the family who had attended previously was not present. We have also used it to find out about what people thought a dead parent, if that person were present now, might say about the difficulties that a family was facing. On occasion, when someone with intellectual disabilities does seem to have difficulty with questions about an absent member's point of view, we adapt the question to, "What *did* Tom say?" or even, "What *does* Tom say?" We can then begin to ask questions about differences between views.

Metaphor

The use of metaphors can, in our experience, be particularly helpful in facilitating conversations with people with intellectual disabilities. We have made much use of metaphor and story telling in talking and thinking about the material that clients bring. We base these conversations on the practices of narrative therapy (White, 1984; White & Epston, 1990b; Epston, White, & Murray, 1992) (see also Scior & Lynggaard, chapter 6). Using these ideas we have found that events that were previously neglected in our conversations with families, events that contradicted the problem-saturated description of life, have had the chance to emerge and be considered. For example, we had been working with Larry, a young adult with mild intellectual disabilities, and his family for about a year. A psychiatrist referred Larry for aggressive behaviours towards his parents such as spitting, throwing things, and shouting. Although we initially tried to open up a conversation with the family about this, we found ourselves working for several months on issues of independence, communication, and relationships. They seemed to find this useful, sharing with us successes that they had had in changing their behaviour. However, when periodically we would ask about the aggressive behaviours, we always got the same response: the behaviours were continuing, no better, no worse, and Larry did not act like this when at his job at the supermarket. The conversation around this topic would then grind to a halt.

After nearly a year of meeting, Larry opened up the session by saying that he was not himself. We wondered who he was and asked him. This opened up a rich discussion about Larry's externalization of his aggressive behaviours. He said that sometimes he was kind, cooperative, and helpful. We asked what we should call this, and he said, "Nice Larry". He then said sometimes he would spit and curse and that we should call this "Evil Larry". We asked about different circumstances where "Evil Larry" or "Nice Larry" would be around, and he said that "Evil Larry" did not come out at work because of the "Lemurs". He went on to elaborate, describing three toy lemurs that he had in his bedroom and that he carried around with him in his head to stop "Evil Larry" from coming out at work. We went on to discuss the special powers that each lemur had (one was fast, another was strong), how and when they could use these powers to help "Nice Larry" and stop "Evil Larry", and what help he may like from his parents in helping to win the "battle". He also kept a scorecard noting each time either "Nice Larry" emerged or "Evil Larry" won out. The use of a metaphor taken from Larry's ideas enabled us to have a different and more useful conversation with him and his family about how they might think about the aggressive behaviour and how they might respond to it in a more helpful way.

* * *

In our work with another family, the elaboration of references to characters in the popular British television BBC serial drama *EastEnders* proved helpful. This is an extract from our second session with the Ellis family. Alan, an adult with intellectual disabilities, is talking with Denise, the lead practitioner, and his father (Brian) and mother (Marjorie):

> *Alan:* "Can I say another thing?"
>
> *Denise:* "Of course."
>
> *Alan:* "I know it's not normal what I'm doing—staying up in the middle of the night [*sad tone*] ... um ... I'll just spit this out ... right ... I know we had a good time on holiday—no barneys or anything ... you [*father*] always make noises like Phil Mitchell [*character from* EastEnders] all the time ..." [*Pause for 2 seconds.*]

At this point we had ideas of violence, aggression, shouting, and so forth but made no comment based upon these assumptions.

> *Alan:* "Why ... why ... do you do it all the time, making noises like Phil Mitchell ..." [*Pause for 2 seconds.*]
>
> *Brian:* "Because none of us are perfect ... that includes you ..." [*Pause*]
>
> *Alan:* "Mum, don't do it, why do you do it? ..." [*5-second pause.*]
>
> *Brian:* "What annoys me is you do it all the time."
>
> *Denise:* "What sort of noises do you mean?"
>
> *Brian:* "Clearing the throat." [*Cough.*]

There then followed a lengthy and angry-sounding fast-paced conversation about who coughs the most/the loudest/the longest in the family and different ideas about why that was so.

* * *

Each time we reflect upon this conversation, new ideas come into mind. For example, as Alan had brought the *EastEnders* theme to the conversation as a metaphor for what his father was doing, we wondered if we could use this as a different way of exploring family relationships. For example, we wondered which character each member of the family thought he or she was and the meaning of this. We wondered which character they might choose to be, the meaning of this, and how this might help them have a different conversation about what was going on for them and to perhaps do things differently in the future. We thought about exploring these ideas through role-play and swapping roles to gain new perspectives. The Ellis family were unable to attend their next session with us, so there was a long gap between this session and their third session. They did not bring the *EastEnders* theme as a metaphor to this third session; they wanted to talk about other issues. We responded to this by listening to their new ideas (their feedback) rather than privileging our "expert" ideas about the continuing use of the *EastEnders* metaphor.

Example from practice

We end this chapter by describing our work with Anna, who was part of a complex system involving various professionals and family members. This example illustrates how a person categorized as having moderate to severe intellectual disabilities and severe communication problems might begin to participate in a systemic process. It also illustrates our attempts at working more collaboratively rather than hierarchically, trying to set a context for change rather than being too directive, and demonstrates the use of genograms to facilitate the expression of ideas. By convening the important people in Anna's life and by facilitating a conversation, a context was created where, for the first time, she could begin to co-create ideas with the important people in her life about the meaning of her relationships with them. This is a description of the first session with Anna, her family, and the professional system.

Referral

Anna was referred to the team by Ellie, her social worker. Ellie requested help for Anna's residential carers and day staff in devising a consistent approach for working with Anna. Ellie's concern was that Anna was becoming "too fond" of her female residential carers and that, consequently, Anna was very distressed when the carers finished their shifts. Ellie also told us that it had been decided in a meeting that all staff should refrain from any physical contact with Anna (i.e., cuddling, kissing, touching) unless it was necessary to help with activities of daily living. We heard several different views about this decision.

Judith, Anna's keyworker from the adult day centre, thought this was a good idea as Anna would not get "too close" to staff and "suffer unnecessary heartache". On the other hand, Alice, one of Anna's residential staff, had expressed her misgivings about professionals prescribing that Anna could not have physical contact from them, stating that this was quite inappropriate and might be an infringement of her human rights.

Convening and pre-session working hypothesis

For the first meeting we invited Anna, Brenda (Anna's cousin), Ellie (Anna's social worker), Judith (Anna's keyworker from the day centre), Clare (Anna's speech and language therapist), and Alice (residential care staff). Denise was the lead practitioner, and two of her colleagues formed the reflecting team. In the team's discussion before the session, we wondered if Anna felt confused and distressed by the mixed messages about physical contact and intimacy that she received from the various people in her life. Our concerns for the residential staff, the day-centre staff, and the cousin were that they each felt misunderstood by the others and frustrated that their views were not being heard or put into practice. The reason for the referral was that everyone in the system "felt stuck" and did not know how to move forward.

In our pre-session meeting, the team and the lead practitioner devised the following questions as guides to the meeting: "I have asked you all to come today, and I was wondering what your ideas were about that?" "Who thought it was a good idea, who next?" "Who is not here today, and if they were here what would they think about this referral?" "What ideas did you have about the sorts of things we could talk about today?" The referral stated that Anna had no verbal communication, only "*la*" for yes and "*n*" for no, but she had pretty good comprehension. Thus, we were wondering if she would be able to understand these questions or respond to them. We thought that perhaps we would ask her to do a relationship map in the session, possibly with the help of the other participants. This, we thought, might make her feel engaged in the session and introduce the context of her various relationships, particularly since the referral concerned what her different relationships meant to her.

Focus of session

The focus of the session was the participants' shared wish that they wanted Anna to be happy and that they each would feel awful if they believed that Anna was deprived of the appropriate physical contact. Initially in the session, the following beliefs were expressed. Alice wanted the session to involve listening and learning. Her hope was that we would come up with some appropriate guidelines for Anna's carers around touching her. Judith described how she felt it was difficult for Anna to cope when carers finished shifts. Brenda felt that she was concerned for Anna's happiness and that she would hate to feel that Anna was deprived of kisses and cuddles, since "Feeling loved is the basis for life". She did not express any explicit views about the goals of our session, but implied that thinking about Anna's happiness would be enough. Ellie had looked into her professional codes of conduct in respect of physical contact between carers and clients and felt that they were, "Grey and fluid, and based on an element of trust". She hoped that our session would help establish guidelines on how physically to interact with Anna, while not depriving her of affection. She also hoped our session would shed light on whether Anna was capable of making choices like a "child" or like a "woman."

Use of relationship map

At this point we invited Anna to create a relationship map by asking her, "Who is important to you?" She named various people with the help of her electronic communication aid, photograph book, and the other participants in the session. Denise wrote each name on flip-chart paper, and Anna told her where to place the names. Through this process Anna was able to share her ideas about who was important to her. This surprised some of the people present, as Anna's ideas were different from their ideas about Anna's ideas.

Co-creating the conversation

After hearing some of Anna's ideas through the creation of the relationship map, we decided to create a context whereby Anna could have further opportunities and time to voice her view in relation to the others present. We explored with Anna, through the use of an individualized system of ranking difference, who she liked and disliked. She used her communication book with photographs and the map created earlier to show us people she knew. She chose seven photographs of people and paired them up with the Makaton symbols for "like", "love", and "hate". She did not choose the "love" symbol for anyone. She showed us that she "liked" her carers, her brother, and three friends by choosing the "like" symbol and saying *"la"* ["yes"]. She showed us that she "hated" two men from the day centre, showing us the symbol for "noisy".

Anna raised some interesting differences between her views and the views of the others present. First, all of the participants had different ideas to Anna about whom they thought she would say were her friends (they did not identify the same three friends that Anna had chosen). There followed a conversation between the carers and Anna. Carers from the home and the day centre heard from Anna about whom she liked at the centre. This resulted in arrangements for these friends to be invited to Anna's home for tea. Second, none of the participants anticipated that Anna might express the view that she "hated" somebody. They expressed their surprise in statements such as "I never realized . . . I thought you liked him" and so on, which again prompted further discussion and changes in the meaning previously ascribed to Anna's behaviour. Arrangements were made for Anna to have her meals at the centre with a different, quieter group. Finally, when the day carer chose the "love" symbol for how she thought Anna felt about her home carers, Anna shook her head and said *"n"* ["no"] and gave her the "like" symbol. Following this meeting, the group decided that they could take things forward together without further help from our service.

* * *

While we have left out some of the discussions we had in the session with Anna's carers and the comments from the reflecting team, we think readers will have heard of many similar referrals where there are many different views about "what is best" for the client and the clients' view is not "heard". This example, we hope, helps to demonstrate some ways that systemic ideas may be translated into practice and show that even though someone may be described as having severe intellectual and communication disabilities, he or she may be engaged in a systemic process and helped to find a voice that others can hear.

Conclusion

The aim of this chapter was to highlight some of the ways by which a person with intellectual disabilities might be engaged in a systemic therapeutic process. We hope that systemic practitioners who are unfamiliar with this client group might give consideration to extending their practice to also work with people with intellectual disabilities. This could be done by exploring ideas such as the pace and style of therapy and modifying some techniques such as the use of circular questions. We also hope that clinical psychologists and other practitioners specializing in work with people with intellectual disabilities might consider systemic approaches in their practice. Practices might include convening wider systems of concern (Lang & McAdam, 1995) with the use of a novel space or different location. Also, we recommend paying close attention to clients' feedback and adopting a position of curiosity. Finally, we hope that practitioners might give more consideration to the assumptions and theories that they bring to practice with people with intellectual disabilities.

CHAPTER SIX

New stories of intellectual disabilities: a narrative approach

Katrina Scior and Henrik Lynggaard

The ideas and descriptions of practice presented in this chapter relate to our work as clinical psychologists in two different multidisciplinary community teams for people with intellectual disabilities. While our teams are different in many ways, we both work in large inner-city areas with ethnically and socially diverse populations. We approach our work from the premise that we need to pay close attention to context—be that the context of our clients, our own context, or the social, cultural, and political contexts that shape all our lives. We also believe that a key part of our role as practitioners should be to offer our skills towards empowering people with intellectual disabilities, who, as a group, have long been marginalized, not least through many professional discourses and practices. It was from this premise that we became excited about narrative therapy (White & Epston, 1990). We were particularly attracted to the way that narrative theory and practice attempt to situate problems in a broader social context and question taken-for-granted "realities" and practices. Moreover, we felt an immediate appeal of White and Epston's (1990) premise that we live our lives according to the stories we tell ourselves and the stories we are told by others, and that people do not usually step outside these dominant stories. These ideas resonated with our experience of working with people with intellectual disabilities and their families and carers. We were mindful that problem-saturated stories can have an amazing longevity in this context and that it can be difficult for all to recognize and remember abilities and resources, rather than being overwhelmed with problems and barriers to change. Consequently, narrative therapy's invitation to perceive people as separate from their problems and to give them a voice in constructing preferred stories about themselves and their futures seemed both relevant and promising.

* * *

At the time of writing this chapter, little had been written about narrative therapy with people with intellectual disabilities. We therefore begin by outlining some of the key ideas and practices of narrative therapy and then consider what opportunities narrative therapy may offer in therapeutic work with adults with intellectual disabilities. We conclude the chapter by addressing some questions that the reader might have about using this approach and offer some personal reflections on the effects of incorporating narrative therapy into our own work. The focus here is on adults, not children, with intellectual disabilities, for the simple reason that there is a considerable body of literature on narrative therapy with children and adolescents. By contrast, we have been able to locate only a few papers on the use of narrative therapy with adults with intellectual disabilities (Clare & Grant, 1994; Perry & Gentle, 1997; Lynggaard & Scior, 2002; Matthews & Gates, 2003; Wilcox & Whittington, 2003; Matthews & Matthews, 2005).

What is narrative therapy?

In this section we intend to provide a brief overview of the key theoretical ideas and practices in narrative therapy. These are illustrated in more detail in the next sections with the help of examples from practice. Our account is by no means meant to be exhaustive, and interested readers are advised to refer to excellent overviews by White and Epston (1990), Freedman and Combs (1996), and Morgan (2000).

Multiple influences

Narrative therapy was initially developed by White and Epston (1990) and has evolved from a synthesis of diverse influences. The ideas of various social sciences theorists and poststructuralist philosophers, in particular Foucault, have been instrumental in the development of narrative theory. Foucault wrote extensively on the way that the human subject is shaped and fabricated by societal discourses and practices; in incorporating many of his ideas on knowledge and power, White comes to see therapy as "an inherently political activity, an activity and set of practices inscribed by power relations" (quoted in Besley, 2001, p. 78). Narrative therapy can be situated within a collection of theories that are broadly referred to as postmodern. These theories share a particular way of viewing the world. As such they start from the premise that there is no objective reality out there waiting to be discovered (von Glaserfeld, 1987). In line with poststructuralist ideas, narrative therapy rejects theories and practices that posit underlying, hidden *structures* or forces such as human nature or the unconscious and that often invite the therapist to become an expert who reveals and uncovers "pathology" or the "truth".

* * *

In its theoretical orientation, narrative therapy further shares the social constructionist premise that people's identities are not stable and singular, but fluid and changeable according to context. Reality is seen to be constructed, or "co-created", between individuals through language—that is, it is the communication between people about objects and events that gives them meaning, rather than the objects or events somehow inherently carrying that meaning themselves (Freedman & Combs, 1996). Thus the co-creation of meaning is a *social* process, which is active and ongoing. Social constructionism recognizes that different versions of reality, while equally valid, have different consequences for individuals in the world, with some being more useful than others. Arising from the notion that reality is co-constructed and changeable, social constructionism encourages us to look critically upon taken-for-granted knowledges. In the therapeutic context, this involves questioning what is constructed as "normal" or a "problem" and, in turn, how such constructions were arrived at.

In its practice and development, narrative therapy has links with family therapy and those therapies that pay particular attention to the importance of interaction, context, and the social construction of meaning. Campbell (2003) highlights the influence of the anthropologist Bateson on White and Epston's early writings, in which they place emphasis on families-as-meaning-making systems. The Milan school of systemic therapy also influenced the development of narrative therapy, and Campbell shows that many of the practices of narrative therapy can be viewed as creative variations and extensions of the Milan group's early ideas. However, as Tomm (1998) points out, narrative therapy has shifted "away from a focus on interaction patterns within families per se, to a focus on the effects of cultural beliefs and practices on interactions among family members" (p. 409). This shift has led some to conclude that narrative therapy has moved away from systemic principles and that it has marginalized family experience in favour of a return to an emphasis on individual human psychology (Minuchin, 1998). Narrative therapists have, in turn, emphasized that individuals learn in multiple contexts, not just in an idealized nuclear family, and that there is therefore a need to look more widely for factors that may contribute to difficulties (Combs & Freedman, 1998, p. 407).

The narrative metaphor

As noted, White and Epston (1990) propose that we make sense of our experiences in terms of "stories" or "narratives" that we construct about ourselves and our lives. Using the term "stories" by no means has to imply elaborate and articulate accounts; rather, it refers to ideas we hold about ourselves that come to shape the way we organize our lives and approach new experiences. White and Epston (1990) stress that most of us have multiple stories available to us about ourselves, other people, and our relationships. Some of these stories promote competence and well-being, whereas others serve to constrain, impoverish, or pathologize ourselves. The stories we live and tell ourselves guide how we think, feel, act, and attribute meaning to new experiences. When problem-saturated stories prevail, we are repeatedly invited into disappointment and misery. In practice, narrative therapists attempt to identify exceptions and discrepancies within problem-dominated stories to make space for the emergence of more enabling stories.

Narrative therapy
and people with intellectual disabilities

People who are defined as having intellectual disabilities constitute a wide and diverse group comprising persons who may need 24-hour care to those who can manage on their own or with limited support. Narrative therapy's challenge of dominant discourses and taken-for-granted realities (White, 1991) makes it an appealing approach for therapeutic work with people who collectively have been marginalized and stigmatized like few others. The very word "dis-ability", with its focus on *absence* of "ability", derives from powerful assumptions as to what should be privileged. The focus in narrative therapy on resurrecting and discovering people's abilities and resources, rather than on diagnosing pathology, holds potential promise for working with a group of people who have been largely defined in terms of their limitations and lack of abilities. Moreover, rather than look at people with intellectual disabilities merely as individuals who are largely divorced from the wider context, a narrative approach allows the practitioner to bring cultural and political realities into the room and to open space for marginalized perspectives (White, 1991). Conversations that seek to deconstruct dominant ideas may take place at many different levels: with an individual, with a team of carers, or within an organization.

* * *

It is our experience that problems often get located inside the person with intellectual disabilities, overshadowing or obscuring their abilities and competences. For individuals used to being viewed as "the problem", being invited to put the problem, and not themselves, on the spot through the practice of *externalizing conversations* can be liberating and can relieve the pressure of blame. By considering in detail what effects dominant stories have on the person's view of self and his or her relationships, space is created with the potential to notice other possibilities and choices.

Externalizing conversations

The intention of engaging in externalizing conversations (White & Epston, 1990) is to locate problems in the context of people's lives rather than as an inherent part of them. Through conversations the problem is located as separate and external to the person. This, in turn, can free the person up to view the problem and themselves differently and begin to shape new possibilities.

* * *

In moving on to outline how narrative therapy may be used with people with intellectual disabilities and their families and carers, we draw on Roth and Epston's (1995) framework for externalizing conversations, which we have found helpful. To give the reader an overview of the methods and techniques of an externalizing conversation, we shall cover the following aspects:

- Mapping the influence of the problem on the person's life and relationships
- Recruitment into problem-saturated views of self
- Identifying unique outcomes
- Thickening of new stories
- Consolidating and extending new stories

We hope that the practical examples given throughout illustrate how narrative therapy can offer new avenues of exploration and ways of working with people with intellectual disabilities and those around them.

* * *

As already stated, when people with intellectual disabilities are referred, or come to therapy, they may have spent a lifetime subjected to discourses that perceive them as "the problem". Rather than reinforce negative reputations, such as "Robert *is* angry" or "Sarah *is* depressed", we aim from the outset to rephrase such descriptions in externalizing language—for example, "Sarah struggles with depression". In negotiating a way of talking about the problem, it is obviously crucial that this fits with the meaning and experience of the person whose life the problem is affecting.

The following extract is taken from work with Robert, a 21-year-old man with moderate intellectual disabilities. We (Katrina Scior and team) had been working with Robert's family for some time, when his father died rather suddenly. Over the coming weeks, his mother became increasingly worried about Robert's behaviour and told us that he appeared very angry and had broken objects in the home. He had resisted all her attempts to talk, and she asked us for help to allow Robert to "vent his feelings". We discussed this idea at some length, wondering why it would be more useful for us, rather than for his mother, to have such a conversation with Robert. With both their agreement, we talked with Robert alone, before being joined again by his mother. The following conversation was influenced by Fredman's (1997) inspiring account of work with children and families who have been bereaved.

Katrina: "What are these feelings like, which are not so okay?"

Robert: "A bit down all the time."

Katrina: "Mmm. What is that like?"

Robert: "My dad's gone, hurt inside, hurt is everywhere."

Katrina: "Do you have these feelings right now?"

Robert: "Always the same."

Katrina: "Do they have a name?"

Robert: "Down ones."

To facilitate therapeutic conversations, we have at times found it helpful to make the problem description more concrete by using gestures and drawings—for example, to demonstrate the size of "down ones". Such concrete demonstrations can also be used at a later stage to explore the person's effect on the problem, such as how they may influence and control the problem. Mark, who used to hit his face several times a day, found new momentum in reducing self-hitting in his life when we (Henrik Lynggaard [HL] and Mark) began to chart his progress on a long line that had "hitting myself every day" at one end and "not hitting myself any more" at the other. During every meeting I (HL) would ask Mark where on this line he placed himself now and where he would like to get to. In the course of conversations over several months, Mark moved gradually further and further in his preferred direction of "not hitting myself any more". Together we would trace in detail what abilities and resources had allowed Mark to achieve movements along this line. The visual representation of progress appeared particularly meaningful for Mark, who enjoyed seeing what he was achieving.

Mapping the influence of the problem on the person's life and relationships

In externalizing conversations the practitioner asks in great detail about the problem's effects on a person's actions, relationships, and views of self. The therapeutic intent of such detailed mapping is two-fold: to ensure that the person feels that the practitioner understands his or her experiences; and to enable the person to know it in a different way and gain a more detailed perspective on the problem's effects on his or her life.

So, returning to the example of Robert, once his preferred way of talking about the problem was identified, we began to explore the influence of "down ones" on Robert in more detail.

> *Katrina:* "Are there times when down ones get bigger?"
>
> *Robert* [*sniggers at name*]: "Came when Dad died, has been getting more."
>
> *Katrina:* "What do down ones make you do when they're big?"
>
> *Robert:* "Make me angry. Smash the window."
>
> *Katrina:* "So down ones make you get angry and smash the window. Is that how you want things to be, or do you want them to be different?"

Robert thought about this question for a while. He told us that his mother had taken him to see a doctor, who had given him tablets to calm him down. When we examined the origin of this story of himself as someone with an "anger problem" who needs medication to "calm down", Robert suggested that he had every reason to be angry and that it must be okay to get angry at times. He added that he wanted to have times, though, when he could remember his father and talk about him without "down ones" making him smash things.

Narrative therapy stresses that we should not assume that those we work with share our perceptions of what is problematic or needs changing. Thus we are reminded to always ask about the person's preferred way of living, by asking questions such as "Is that something that suits you?" "Is that a good thing, or a bad thing, or an okay thing to have in your life?" "Can you tell me why?" In our experience the very act of asking such questions results in clients literally sitting up. Although responses mostly are in the form of, "Of course, I don't want anger/anxiety/depression around in my life", we have repeatedly noticed that the question opens room for thinking and discussion, including consideration of what the effect of the problem's disappearance might be.

Recruitment into problem-saturated views of self

Another important aspect of this initial stage of narrative therapy is tracing the history of the problem and exploring how the person was recruited into the problem-saturated view of self. In this process the broader social context can be woven into the conversation, and the effects of taken-for-granted notions such as "disability", "gender", or "failure" can be examined. Although tracing the history of the presenting concern or problem may usually form part of the initial phases of therapy, exploration of the construction and effects of dominant and constraining beliefs is not confined to any one "stage" of therapy as the following example demonstrates. In fact, it has been our experience that attempts to deconstruct beliefs before the person has had an opportunity to have his or her stories witnessed can result in the person not feeling listened to.

Ms Thomas initially sought help because of the erratic sleep pattern of her son, who had profound intellectual disabilities and for whom she had cared more or less singled-handedly for the past twenty-five years. Over the course of a number of conversations she repeatedly described herself as a "useless mother" for not being able to manage her son's complex needs without resorting to help. She felt convinced that her own deceased mother, neighbours, and other women would judge her negatively for not coping better. Gradually we (HL and Ms Thomas) began to explore where these ideas of "always coping, perfect mothers" came from. Who and what generated and supported these ideas of motherhood? Who might be advantaged or disadvantaged by trying to adopt and live by these rules? Ms Thomas explained that guilt at giving birth to a disabled child had triggered her into believing that she had to work doubly hard at being a perfect, coping mother. In talking about these ideas she started noticing that none of the images and stories that were circulated about "how to be a perfect mother" ever included mothers of disabled children. This discovery was enormously liberating for Ms Thomas, who felt she had been recruited into living according to a set of "crazy" rules that had driven her to utter exhaustion and trapped both her and her son.

Identifying unique outcomes

In the process of mapping the influence of the problem on the person, we try to listen out for actions and intentions that do not fit within the dominant, problem-saturated story. Morgan (2000) argues that "a problem will never be 100% successful in claiming a person's life. There will always be exceptions or times of difference" (p. 58). These exceptions are also referred to as unique outcomes (White, 1989) and may tell us about unrecognized abilities, as illustrated in the following brief extract, again from work with Robert.

> *Katrina:* "I am interested in times when you can make down ones smaller or even go away altogether."
> *Robert:* "Okay when I go out."
> *Katrina :* "So there are times when you can make down ones disappear, like when you go out?"
> *Robert:* "Watching my favourite programme, down ones [*again sniggers at name*] go away."
> *Katrina:* "That's interesting! So you can make down ones go away when you go out and when you watch your favourite programme."
> *Robert:* "Yeah."
> *Katrina:* "Is that something you want to do more of or not?"
> *Robert:* "Yeah, feels good."

The identification of unique outcomes is something the narrative therapist is particularly alert to, as clients may not notice these different moments of lived experience and the potential for change they may hold. However, as White (1991) notes, for an event to comprise a unique outcome, the person must be invited to evaluate its significance and judge it as a preferred outcome. In other words, it is important that practitioners distinguish between what they themselves consider a desirable development and what the person who consults them considers an important change. In the process of therapeutic practice, unique outcomes are the building blocks that can constitute the foundation on which new, preferred stories are gradually developed.

Thickening of new stories

When people struggle with difficulties over a long time, it can profoundly affect how they view themselves and can obscure resources and previous accomplishments. For people with intellectual disabilities, stories that describe them as weak and lacking in abilities are often so powerful and prevalent that it may be difficult to construct, live, and circulate alternative stories: stories that speak of abilities, competence, and intentions. The narrative practitioner deliberately seeks to address these areas. Percy (1999) notes: "I view the exploration of such abilities and talents as accessing different identities which may lead to a fuller recognition of certain well-developed attributes the person already possesses—attributes that may be used to defeat or reduce the problem" (p. 33).

In the following extract, the practitioner aims to thicken descriptions of Najeeb as someone who is competent and who can show strength and determination, away from the dominant story of himself as "weak" and "a failure". Najeeb was an 18-year-old man with mild intellectual disabilities whose life had been dominated by rituals. Initial meetings had focused on the effect "stress" (as Najeeb termed the problem) had on him, his relationships, and his view of self. Stress had convinced him that he was "weak", "a failure", and "no good as a person" and that he had no control over the problem whatsoever.

> Henrik: "So how did you go about not letting stress try to make you stay in the house?"
>
> Najeeb: "I don't know. [*After a little pause*] Well, it is not too hard in the daytime. [*Faintly*] I think I'm getting a bit stronger."
>
> Henrik: "I'm sorry? You think what?"
>
> Najeeb [*slightly louder*]: "I think I'm getting a bit stronger."
>
> Henrik: "You're getting stronger! Has anyone else noticed that you are getting stronger?"
>
> Najeeb [*hesitates for a while*]: "People at college. People who used to think that I was quiet."

Henrik: "The people who used to think they could call you names and give you a hard time?"

Najeeb: "Yeah, yeah, them."

Henrik: "And what happened?"

Najeeb: "Well, I shouted at them. I answered back."

Henrik: " What did they do? Did they look surprised?"

Najeeb [*with a faint smile*]: "Yes, they did."

Henrik: "So you can stand up to the people who give you a hard time and surprise them. What does that tell you about yourself?"

Najeeb: "Uhm . . . that I can be strong."

Henrik: "Is that a good thing, being strong?"

Najeeb: "Well, of course."

Moments such as these are extensively elaborated in narrative work, both in terms of detailed description of what exactly happened (known as *elaboration in the landscape of action*) and in terms of their implications for a different perception of self (known as *elaboration in the landscape of identity*) (Morgan, 2002). The therapeutic intention is to develop thin descriptions of change into thicker descriptions by exploring the meaning of the unique outcomes from a number of different perspectives. It is important, however, that the elaboration of new preferred stories is not confined merely to listing personal internal attributes or qualities. Carey and Russell (2003) observe that the pursuit of questions in a single domain can lead to the practitioner getting stuck. "We are interested in exploring the intentions, hopes, values and commitments that shape people's actions rather than any deficits or deficiencies, or for that matter any internal 'resources', 'strengths' or 'qualities'" (Carey & Russell, p. 65). Alice Morgan (2000) provides many examples of questions that access these different domains, and that help in further richly describing and connecting preferred developments.

Consolidating and extending new stories

A key concern of any therapeutic approach is how change is maintained outside the therapeutic setting. Narrative therapy addresses this concern in a number of interesting ways, ways that may be particularly helpful for people who can be very dependent on others in many aspects of their lives. In addition to mapping out the preferred story in great detail in terms of what it means for the person's life, his or her actions and relationships, attention is paid to extending the performance of this alternative story. A range of practices have been described to consolidate and strengthen therapeutic gains. The ones we have found most useful in our work with people with intellectual disabilities and their systems are outlined below. Other creative practices are described in detail by Morgan (2000).

1. *Recruiting an audience.* This describes a practice where significant members of the person's social network are invited to witness the new self-narrative. Roth and Epston (1995) note that the inclusion of others in the newly developing story is essential to anchor and continue the development of the alternative story. In Robert's case, his mother was invited. She not only listened to Robert's developing story as someone who could put anger in its place, but also considered with him how he could extend this new story into the future and find times when he could remember his father without anger taking over.

With Paul, a 59-year-old man with moderate intellectual disabilities, who had been referred because of an "excessive grief reaction" [sic] following the death of William, his friend of thirty years, we (HL and Paul) invited his residential and day-centre keyworkers to join us in the latter stages of the work. Through words, photographs, and drawings, Paul told his keyworkers about the history of his long and close friendship with William. As a result there were now many more people who could join Paul in conversations about William, and sadness no longer stopped Paul from doing the things he had previously enjoyed.

We have learnt that it is important to prepare well when inviting other people to join ongoing work and to have clear ideas about their purpose. Otherwise there is a danger that the person is overwhelmed yet again by problem-saturated descriptions. Where it proves impossible or inappropriate to recruit outside witnesses, the client can be asked to be an audience to his or her new story, by seeing him/herself through the eyes of others. This is done by asking questions such as "What does this tell your Mum about you?" "Who would not be surprised that you have made these changes?" With individuals who may find it very difficult to adopt others' perspectives, we have found that using puppets or dolls can be a useful technique. This allows the performing of the new story and direct observation from the perspective of important members of the person's system.

2. *Use of video and literary means to document and celebrate new knowledges and practices.* Towards the end of our work together, Paul and I (HL) asked another therapist to interview us on video about the work we had done over the previous months. The video became a record that could be used for many purposes: when Paul wanted people who supported him to know something about his friend William; when he wanted to remember something about the "journey" he had travelled; and when, participating in training events, he agreed to show others extracts that illustrated what he had contributed towards the therapist's learning. While many therapeutic approaches will acknowledge how theory is shaped by learning from clients, narrative practitioners will often talk explicitly with clients about how their conversations together have contributed to the practitioner's thinking and work practices. Openly acknowledging that the therapeutic conversation is at least a two-way process can in itself create change. One person I (HL) worked with left the room confidently stating "I teach you too".

From time to time we write letters to the people we are working with, summarizing some of our conversations and documenting achievements. Where a person is reliant on others for reading letters, we always check beforehand if we can send a letter and we sometimes write the letter together. Writing a letter that has several simultaneous audiences can, in our experience, be very powerful. Peter's keyworker, for example, told us that our letters about Peter's courageous struggle with anger had helped her to notice his determination and persistence, where previously she had only seen limitations and "challenging behaviour". For detailed examples of the use of "therapeutic letters", readers are encouraged to see White and Epston (1990), Freeman, Epston, and Lobovits (1997), and Fox (2003).

3. *Asking the person to share the new understanding with others.* In our work, we often invite the person to share their knowledge with others—for example, through questions such as: "I sometimes meet with other people like yourself who really struggle to get one up on stress: are there any tips you want to share with them?" We have noticed that in addition to strengthening the new story, this can have an empowering effect on people who rarely have "knowledge" attributed to them or are asked to share it with others.

Constraints of the approach

Readers may well be left with questions about some apparent limitations of drawing on a narrative-therapy approach when working with people with intellectual disabilities. In this final section we aim to address some of these. First, we are mindful that the examples cited in this chapter tell stories of people with mild and moderate intellectual disabilities. Based on our experience, we find no greater obstacles in making this approach accessible to people with mild and moderate intellectual disabilities than is the case with other language-based therapeutic approaches. In direct work with people, the pace of conversations and the pace of the work may, of course, proceed at a slower rate than with people who do not have intellectual disabilities. Questions may need to be repeated and concepts unpacked. But as long as language is kept fairly concrete and simple, drawings and pictures are used where appropriate, and the practitioner frequently checks mutual understanding, there is scope for engaging in useful conversations and interactions. Indeed, the emphasis in narrative therapy on avoiding the language of disorder and diagnostic labels in favour of naming difficulties in terms of what they mean to people's lives seems to be helpful in engaging people with intellectual disabilities. We are, however, aware that in some writings on narrative therapy questions are suggested that may appear very complicated. It has been our experience, in watching the therapeutic conversations of many eminent narrative practitioners, that they use much more simplified language in their work than may be suggested by condensed versions of questions that appear in theoretical papers. Moreover, from narrative research with people with intellectual disabilities (see Booth & Booth, 1996) and narrative therapy with young children (see Freeman, Epston, & Lobovits, 1997; Morgan, 1999), we can learn how concepts and methods can be made more accessible. Having said that, we are, of course, not advocating narrative therapy as an approach that is suitable for everyone, irrespective of circumstances or preferences.

* * *

Readers may also be wondering about the accessibility of narrative therapy for people with more severe or profound intellectual disabilities. We frequently adopt a narrative approach in working indirectly—for example, by working with families and carers. In this work, we are mindful that the less a person has the means for participating in the construction of meaning, the more that person is subject to others' power to story the person's life for him or her and influence the material conditions of his or her life. This means that for individuals with severe or profound intellectual disabilities, an approach that focuses on stories and beliefs is not irrelevant, even though the conversation partners may not be the individual but people in the wider system. The construct of "challenging behaviour" is one area where the stories that are constructed about the problem have frequently become inseparable from the person and are powerfully influenced by the beliefs and experiences of the story-makers, such as carers and professionals, as well as the broader social context. But we have noticed that as different and less problem-saturated stories begin to be told about the person, different possibilities for actions and interactions begin to open up. For example, in the work with Debbie, a young woman with severe intellectual disabilities and a tendency to spit at people, it was questions that were directed at bringing forth at least a glimpse of a different Debbie that began to create a difference. We asked the staff team questions such as "Could you tell me what you most appreciate about Debbie—it might be something she likes, some particular abilities she has, or something else?" The staff who had known her the longest had no difficulties in mentioning Debbie's joy at hearing or participating in making music. Although foreshortening a longer piece of work, it was talking with the staff about different aspects of Debbie's identities, rather than exclusively focusing on the spitting, that helped create shifts in interactions. Over time, this motivated staff team became interested in exploring other skills that Debbie might possess that they had not previously noticed. It appeared that the staff's closer attention to, and interest in, Debbie's subtle ways of communicating had resulted in more positive interactions where she, in turn, seemed to experience less and less need for behaviours such as spitting. Of course, we are not wanting to give the impression that such work is always straightforward or that narrative approaches make a significant difference in all circumstances.

* * *

On a different note, readers may be concerned about potential ethical dilemmas in helping a person develop stories about "preferred realities", where this person's life options may seem very limited. When we initially began to use narrative ideas in our work, we were apprehensive about the danger of raising false hopes, where the person may have little control over whether a certain problem is in their lives. Narrative theory suggests that even where a person has a genetic or neurological problem, he or she will always have at least a small amount of control. Morgan (1997) argues that it is more valuable to focus on these instances of the person's ability to influence the problem than on all the times when the problem appears to have taken over the person's life. The work of the peer counsellors of the Irish Wheelchair Association (Boyle et al., 2003) may also have relevance to practitioners in the field of intellectual disabilities: the peer counsellors question many taken-for-granted assumptions about disability, and they offer practitioners new ways of responding to the experience of disability. In particular, they remind us that disability is multi-storied and that there can be ways of renegotiating relationships with disability.

* * *

Given that narrative therapy shares the notion that clients, not therapists, are the "experts" on their own lives (Anderson & Goolishian, 1992), some readers may question how they might use their large knowledge base and training to best effect. White (1991) suggests that we can use our ideas and knowledges—what he terms "local knowledge"—as possibilities and negotiate their usefulness with clients. Fredman (1997, 2001) illustrates beautifully how, if invited by those who seek our help, we can contribute psychological theories to the pool of ideas and explore which have a poorer or better fit for the person's lived experience. In these instances, such stories and theories are offered tentatively, not as ultimate truths but as further possibilities. In this process we may well share our knowledge—for example, of aspects of behavioural techniques—with clients and carers.

* * *

Finally, readers may wonder what evidence is available, aside from compelling examples, to suggest that narrative therapy is effective and useful. The rapid expansion of narrative ideas among practitioners in many countries, the prolific growth in publications on the topic, the application of the ideas to different client groups, and the establishment of communities of users (i.e., anti-anorexic league), all in a relatively short time, certainly tell stories of a growing appeal of narrative ideas. To our knowledge, however, there are no published outcome studies or comparative studies that would satisfy the so-called gold standard of randomized control research. However, important and relevant as the question about effectiveness and usefulness may be, we can only approach it by a reminder of the different assumptions underpinning modern and postmodern views of research (Larner, 2004). For narrative practitioners, it has been important to approach the questions of research and evidence in a manner that is coherent with the underlying ethos and principles of narrative therapy (Dulwich Centre Publications, 2004). Michael White (1995), for example, distinguishes between primary and secondary research and asserts that those people who are practicing therapy, along with the persons who seek therapy, are the primary or basic researchers, and those people who collect data in a more formal way are the secondary or supportive researchers. This rethinking on what is commonly understood by research is summarized well by David Epston:

> I have always thought of myself as doing research, but on problems and the relationships that people have with problems, rather than on the people themselves. The structuring of narrative questions and interviews allow me and others to co-research problems and the alternative knowledges that are developed to address them. [Epston, 2001, p. 178; quoted in Dulwich Centre Publications, 2004, p. 30]

As a consequence of these different conceptions of research, the evidence base that is building up within narrative therapy has taken on a different form from research undertaken within a modernist paradigm. Thus the outcome of narrative therapy with people without intellectual disability has been documented over a number of years using a broad range of qualitative research methods (e.g., Besa, 1994; St James-O'Connor, Meakes, Pickering, & Schuman, 1997; Epston, 1999; Hoper, 1999; Sprague, 2000). Other approaches to research are set out in two special issues of the *International Journal of Narrative Therapy and Community Work* (2004, Vols. 2 & 3). One type of research within the narrative school consists of inquiring into the solution knowledges and problem-solving skills of people who are consulting therapists. The solution knowledges that are articulated are documented and compiled in archives so that they can be made available to others who are facing similar difficulties. A particular noteworthy example of this are the archives of the anti-anorexia/bulimia league. According to a note by Epston (1999), the archive was running to some 5,000 pages in 1999! We have no doubt that debates will continue about the evidence base of narrative therapy and the "politics of evidence" (see Larner, 2004) and that there will be many contributions to this debate by people embracing both modern and postmodern perspectives. It is our hope that over time there will also be a growing number of accounts that describe the use of narrative ways of working with people with intellectual disabilities, as well as accounts where the clients' comments on their experiences take central place.

Reflection on our experiences

We hope we have succeeded in illustrating how narrative therapy may be useful in working with people with intellectual disabilities and their wider systems. Narrative therapy invites us to look at people and the world in a different way, and it has certainly encouraged both of us to reflect on our own beliefs and assumptions. Learning about narrative therapy has prompted me (KS) to continually question not only my practice in therapy, but my deeply held ideas about such concepts as "disability" and their meaning in day-to-day life and "professional–client" interactions. It has made us recognize how, as clinical psychologists, we have been trained in many models that focus our eyes on problems, limitations, and deficits yet can blind us to clients' abilities and resources. Many of narrative therapy's premises and techniques can appear so very different from many of the modernist approaches covered in my training that I (KS) am frequently pushed to wonder what the people I work with make of narrative ideas and practices. Of course, the very same should apply to other ideas I draw on in my work (mainly cognitive behavioural therapy), for which positive evidence of their effectiveness with people with intellectual disabilities is only slowly emerging. However, it is perhaps the aspects of narrative therapy that make clients *and* therapists literally *sit up* that prompt such constant questioning and caution, for the very reason that they challenge us to take a very different look at things that have long been taken for granted.

* * *

I (HL) have found that introducing narrative practices into my work has been both inspiring and energizing. In my work with individuals, it has invited me to explore different ways of talking to and being with people. I continue to be amazed at the richness of the ideas and creative practices that have been generated within the international narrative community. The more I work in this way and the more I read, the more layers I discover within the approach and the more possibilities open up; including possibilities for offering something that is, hopefully, more respectful to those with whom I work. Most importantly, the narrative approach values and embraces diversity and promotes a way of relating to others that certainly fits with my preferred way of being in the world.

CHAPTER SEVEN

Supporting transitions

Jennifer Clegg and Susan King

We introduce this chapter by describing the context of our work and the various ways that systemic ideas have affected it. Three systemic ideas inform our transition interventions: "side-step autonomy", "keep multiple realities alive", and "expect engagement and disengagement". These ideas organize the structure of subsequent sections. We summarize the research literature that supports and explains the ideas, some of which may be unfamiliar to professionals working in intellectual disability services. Vignettes illustrate the issues and give some ideas of how we engaged with families or systems seen within our clinic. We conclude by pulling together our thoughts about this work, including some personal reflections.

Our contexts

Our transition into systemic therapists began late in 1997, when we started offering sessions to adults with intellectual disabilities and their carers in a hospital-based clinic and, less formally, in their homes. We are especially grateful to the families and staff who dared to try out an explicitly experimental clinic in its earliest days. Our work has been shaped by training at Leeds and Birmingham, mainly through supervision from Paula Boston and John Burnham; and by support over many years from Mark Pearson.

* * *

We work for Nottinghamshire Healthcare NHS Trust, a large mental health trust. The family therapy clinic is a component of specialist community health services provided to adults with intellectual disabilities within Nottingham's urban population of 640,000. The Trust has been a patient and facilitative host of this new systemic service. Their commitment to the long term was demonstrated by managers freeing clinical time for us to train sequentially over six years, equipping the clinic, and allowing the service to develop without excessive scrutiny. Nottingham's intellectual disability service also fosters that rare thing, a collegial environment: the questions and appreciative feedback of peers created an ideal context in which to develop our understanding of systemic ideas. Nurses, music therapists, and psychiatrists in the service have attended, or are now attending, introductory courses in family therapy, and we hope that this confluence of intellectual disability and family therapy will continue to be fruitful for people who use the services.

The systemic clinic has a one-way screen and a video link and is located within the psychiatric outpatients department in a large general hospital. Access is difficult, parking atrocious. However, it is a relatively neutral space for most service users. Families who have attended the specialist intellectual disability service base for years often say that the many different professionals they have met, and interventions they have experienced, tend to blur. It seems to help if something new, such as family therapy, occurs in a new location, perhaps because it is easier to notice difference in a different place.

A team of up to four members has maintained this clinic for seven years now. Both the authors have been there throughout, along with at least one non-psychologist. Colleagues from psychiatry, social work, and nursing have been members at different times; experiential team-building exercises with them have been important influences on the development of systemic practice in the Nottingham service. For almost all of its history the team has had both genders represented, a factor we consider important to the team's effective functioning. Cultural sensitivity is aided by reflecting on the second author's experiences of migration, by the first author's decade in Scotland, and by histories brought by other team members.

The clinic has changed over time from monthly to fortnightly to weekly; referrals continue to come in spates, only to dry up again. Since the service is unfamiliar to many staff, we explore different aspects of systemic thinking and practice in workshops for them, which run about twice a year. Workshops often result in referrals and in people choosing to attend introductory courses in family therapy. Word-of-mouth between clients, staff, and families is also starting to make a small increase in demand for the service. However, the referral rate drops significantly each time reorganizations occur. In the last seven years we have endured two NHS reorganizations; the division into city and county services of our key partner, social services; and now privatization of intellectual disability services formerly delivered by the NHS and social services, in part influenced by the White Paper *Valuing People* (Department of Health, 2001). Such frequent changes make it hard for potential referrers to remain mindful of any innovation.

The clinic allows us to reflect upon our work and offer one another live supervision, but it is far from being our only site of systemic practice. Sometimes we work with systems individually, consulting with the team about the work. At other times we work as pairs in people's homes, with one person as therapist and the other as note-taker and reflector. Intervening within the professional system is another key to creating a context for systemic practice: to increase the likelihood that colleagues in community teams will view difficulties in systemic terms, we take whatever opportunities present themselves to develop conversations about the importance of relationships and multiple perspectives. This makes it easier to develop solutions that involve rather than ignore issues of relationship.

* * *

We offer systemic consultation to colleagues who feel they are getting mired in complexity; perhaps significantly, we also seek systemic consultation from others when we feel the same way. Standing back to reflect about ways that the service system may be mirroring family issues is often preferable to the sense of failure people can feel when professionals give up and refer on. We discuss whether referring on will generate an impossibly complex service system around an already complex family. In most cases, we assume that the competence to create change resides within the existing family and care system; the task for the practitioner is to facilitate its identification and use. Sometimes we work with staff teams that are experiencing low morale and high sickness. Often these teams have had periods of great enthusiasm and creativity. We set out to hear about that in preference to the history of how their problems started, but we respect their need for us to understand the problems too. One way to engender systemic change is by starting new conversations. Mason's (1991) description of the systemic handover has informed this work.

The last way that systemic ideas have shaped our work concerns practice discussion within the psychology service itself. Seeking new directions for difficult situations tended to entrench a narrative of failure. Since each person had individual clinical supervision to discuss difficulties, we agreed to try presenting successful examples of work during monthly meetings; these do not all involve systemic ways of working, because other colleagues have different specialist skills. In our meetings we consider why a particular approach worked best for that person; what other possible approaches could have been used; and what might help in the future when this person encounters predictable but different hurdles. When rapid change occurs after a brief period of work, we consider how that person became so ready for change and what colleagues or the person concerned have done to facilitate that. Two years on, such discussions have made us more creative about naming one another's qualities and have enlarged our therapeutic range, but we remain mindful of steering between bland self-satisfaction and conversations that make people feel judged or condemned.

* * *

This outline of our context and practices offers a position from which to view the sections that follow. The next section presents three ideas that inform our work with transition.

Three ideas to organize interventions with transition

Clients often encounter difficulty as they move from child to adult services, but other transitions can also challenge systems: when families reconfigure as a new partner enters the home, when the person with intellectual disabilities leaves home, and when people experience bereavement or other losses. Such transitions are stressful for everybody, but many people with intellectual disabilities appear to find adapting to change particularly hard. The following three ideas developed from reflections and debates about the published literature on systemic practice and on intellectual disability. They were selected for potential utility and refined in practice through discussion with clients using a range of different approaches. They are introduced in what follows, but most of the literature on which they are based is discussed later in the chapter, followed by vignettes illustrating their use in practice.

Side-step autonomy

In liberal humanist cultures, the transition to adult services is framed by the expectation that the person will or has already become a fully autonomous adult. Yet a number of contemporary philosophers have observed how difficult people find it to notice the mutual dependencies of contemporary life as we become ill, pregnant, or afraid; when we fly in aeroplanes, take financial advice, grow old; and so forth. Obliterating or ignoring such dependencies puts young people with intellectual disabilities into an untenable position. Exhorting them to assert their adulthood not only focuses on a dimension that is problematic, it also de-emphasizes more salient dimensions of identity. Even though most welcome the news that they are now adult, young people with intellectual disability know that the usual markers of adulthood—a job, a car, a spouse, a child—are a distant hope at best. Moreover, repeatedly stating that they are or soon will be autonomous confuses them and others about how to ask for, or offer, help.

Side-stepping dominant discourses is an important strategy that systemic practitioners use to ensure their conversation is not "more of the same": it makes space for other ideas. Professionals working in intellectual disability services may find the idea of side-stepping autonomy strange, because there are so many injunctions to empower, to avoid patronizing, to enhance the person's adult status. Yet for many clients and carers encountering difficulties, especially at the transition to adult services, the discourse of autonomy leads them up a blind alley. To develop a conversation that does make a difference to people, it is necessary to side-step the dominant idea and develop new ways to conceptualize the situation.

Keep multiple realities alive

The core family therapy idea of keeping multiple realities alive describes the need to hold in mind, and to keep open within therapeutic conversations, a "multiverse" of different possibilities (e.g., Andersen, 1991, especially pp. 38–39). A prime task for systemic practitioners is refusing to "get married" to any single idea—a teasing criticism intended to help us stand back from close association with any particular position. It can be difficult to validate a range of possibilities within the dominant discourse of "values", which have created a culture preoccupied with independence, protection, and traditional gender roles. It can also be difficult to validate a range of possibilities because the uncertainty associated with intellectual disability is uncomfortable. A premature decision for any course of action can look attractive to everybody involved because it creates certainty, however misguided. Yet the systemic practitioner works most effectively when he or she notices and questions those ideas that close down possibilities for creative thinking in different areas.

Expect engagement and disengagement

Whenever a family stops attending sessions without achieving the changes they sought, we reflect about whether we may have misunderstood something important, misjudged the pace, or failed to balance the different needs and demands of all system members. It is common for some family members to want ideas for action while others want emotional validation; practitioners do not always develop ways to meet these different needs. Other families clearly find sitting together in a room unusual and uncomfortable; if we failed to notice and then negotiate a process that was comfortable, disengagement must be expected. Counter-cultural situations presented other hurdles that we have not always enabled people to surmount—for example, men with intellectual disabilities who deeply resent a younger sister taking responsibility for them when their mother falls ill, or second-generation immigrants caught in different gender, age, or family expectations. On the other hand, external events occurred quite frequently that seemed to crush any hope of therapy making a difference: the suicide of a family member; ongoing community harassment; a significant person being or becoming seriously ill. Our (far from random) sample of families has contained much higher levels of physical illness than we had expected. Engagement problems should be expected, since many clients experience multiple problems; also, knowledge about ways to adapt systemic techniques for families with disabled members is in its infancy. Persistence and creativity in developing ways to help people achieve change in their lives are important, but so is remaining open to the possibility that people will need to disengage from time to time. Communicating an understanding of this possibility removes a sense that either they or we have "failed". People should be able to disengage when they need to, and to re-engage when they have enough resources to carry them through the change they seek.

Having presented three key ideas that organize our thinking and our practice with issues of transition, we now turn to reviewing the literature that informs these ideas.

Literature review

Although transition is frequently described as a problem for people with intellectual disabilities, there is virtually no theoretical analysis of why transitions should provoke distress. Explanations generally rest on an implicit "lack-of-practice" notion from normalization: since people with intellectual disabilities live impoverished lives, the assumption is that they merely need a range of ordinary experiences to become able to deal with ordinary life. This contains the unspoken belief that transition problems would be entirely resolved by more experience and improved services. We question this position, by reviewing policy and research about transition, before summarizing research relevant to the three organizing ideas outlined in the previous section.

Transition policy and research

The transition to adult services is one of eleven targets for service improvement in *Valuing People* (Department of Health, 2001). Heslop, Mallett, Simons, and Ward (2002) studied transition planning and services in a sample that ranged from 25-year-olds who had made the transition six years previously in 1994 (in a different policy context) to 13-year-olds who had yet to make it. They criticized transition planning for failing to involve a quarter of the young people in the planning process; for failing to discuss two main concerns of the young people and their carers, employment and housing; and for failing to generate enough options for employment and housing. Clegg, Sheard, Cahill, and Osbeck (2001) describe the different experiences of carers and service providers just after a cohort of school-leavers with severe intellectual disabilities had moved into adult services. The cohort contained almost as many people whose move to services was associated with a reduction in challenging behaviours as those whose difficult childhood behaviours remained. Nevertheless, both carers and providers described themselves as battling to make the other understand them.

Difficulties may occur just as frequently at other life-cycle transitions, but their unpredictability makes them harder to research. Some people fail to make transitions into what are considered to be better environments. While it is generally assumed that the environment did not suit the person, it is equally probable that it was the transition process itself that was too disturbing. Ghaziuddin (1988) reported that half of a sample of adults with intellectual disabilities referred to psychiatric services had experienced a life event in the twelve months previously. Comparing psychiatric hospital admissions in adults with and without disabilities, Stack, Haldipur, and Thompson (1987) found that people with intellectual disabilities were more likely to be admitted when life events involved conflict or loss. In another study of 310 adults with intellectual disabilities seen consecutively in a psychiatric service (Ryan, 1994), 17% had post-traumatic stress disorder.

Why would people with intellectual disabilities be vulnerable to transition-related distress? One explanation is that they have more stressful lives. For example, in mainstream secondary schools in an English city, 59% of children with special needs reported being bullied but only 16% of mainstream children (Whitney, Smith, & Thompson, 1994). Repeated experiences of rejection may make it difficult to trust new environments to be welcoming. Another explanation is that people with intellectual disabilities are more vulnerable to life stress. Cummins (2004) described the robust processes that allow most people to keep their subjective well-being around the normal range of 75%. People with intellectual disabilities are at much greater risk of those homeostatic mechanisms being defeated: they have less control of their environments, are more likely to experience negative life-events, and rarely have the money or relationships most of us use to buffer them.

Fragile systems maintaining subjective well-being are implicated in the way people accommodate major life-events. A third, possibly complementary, explanation is that people with intellectual disabilities appear more likely to react strongly to the losses that are a necessary part of successful transitions. The view that people with intellectual disabilities often make dependent relationships with key people is rarely voiced now, although it was a feature of early twentieth-century medical textbooks. Yet every practitioner knows young people with intellectual disabilities who react when their mother shares attention—for example, kicking her during telephone conversations until she ends them. Some evidence concerning intense relationships comes from Clegg and Lansdall-Welfare's (2003) research review, which argued that people with intellectual disabilities are clearly more vulnerable to bereavement-related distress. Perhaps preoccupation with existing relationships makes it hard for them to let go and move on. Why might that be? Attachment theory considers increased challenging behaviour to be separation protest: it expresses the person's urgent demand to replace or retrieve their secure emotional base. Evidence for this possibility comes from Atkinson et al.'s (1999) data on young children with Down's syndrome, which found significant numbers to be insecurely attached to their main carer and hence vulnerable to attachment disorder on starting primary school. This attachment perspective is elaborated by Clegg and Lansdall-Welfare (1995), Clegg and Sheard (2002), Hill, Fonagy, Safier, and Sargent (2003), and Janssen, Schuengel, and Stolk (2002). Insecure attachment relationships with the main carer limit curiosity and constrain exploration of the world; these are considered key transition-related abilities.

Side-step autonomy

Some practitioners may fear that abandoning the assumption of autonomy patronizes the adult and runs the risk of treating them as a child. Rose (1999), however, warns that humanity is impoverished when ideas of mutuality and commitment to others are dismissed. We invite practitioners to loosen their attachment to autonomy as the dominant idea informing transition to adult services: it sets up unattainable expectations and backs people into an ethical *cul de sac*. This will strike many intellectual disability staff as an odd position, but we are not alone in taking it.

Clinicians such as Skelly (2002) have argued that *Valuing People* (Department of Health, 2001) may be "denial of disability writ large" (p. 45). He noted how frequently staff push clients into placements that require unrealistic levels of independence where they fail, leaving all concerned distressed. Yet nobody performs at the peak of their ability on a long-term basis. Thomas (2001) described the depression that staff experience when they predicate their worth as workers on helping service users with intellectual disabilities to develop as autonomous individuals; this elaborates previous research into staff burnout. She suggests that services are built upon an active denial of disability, to enable staff to maintain optimism and carry on with the work. This breaks down when limits to autonomy are reached, and staff descend into hopelessness. Thomas recommends that services shift their success criteria in order to continue working with people with intellectual disabilities without denying that there are limitations to their autonomy. There is support from philosophy, too. Reinders (2000) argues that the assertion of autonomous self-hood rests on liberal morality, which treats people without autonomy as either potential persons or as non-persons. To ensure they are treated as persons, liberal convention has developed the unsustainable fiction that all people with intellectual disability are autonomous, or, if not, they could be if everybody around them tried hard enough. When this clearly fails to apply to individuals with the greatest disabilities, exponents insist that they should be treated *as if* they are autonomous despite clear evidence to the contrary. This wards off the feared implications of becoming a non-person in liberal culture. Reinders argues for an alternative ethical stance, hermeneutics, which theorizes interdependence rather than dependence and values humans not for what they can do, but for what they are. The implications for practice of this alternative conceptualization have been described in a review of bereavement (Clegg & Lansdall-Welfare, 2003) and of services for offenders (Clegg, 2004).

Keep multiple realities alive

This core idea from family therapy (Goldner, 1998) is challenging for intellectual disability services in which meaning is difficult to create and easily dissolved. Stolk and Kars (2000) found almost a quarter of their sample of parents whose child had profound intellectual disabilities discussed having had doubts about the purpose of their child's life at times. Perhaps avoidance of that thought provides one reason why intellectual disability services repeatedly believe they have found the magic answer (Potts & Howard, 1986), rejecting much that went before: hopes invested in psychiatry were quickly transferred to behaviourism, normalization, and then community care. More recently Holborn and Vietze (1998) implied that person-centred planning (PCP) is the latest incarnation of the magic answer, arguing that a spirit of alchemy seems to be evoked when governments imagine that PCP can turn poorly funded services made of lead into gold. Taking a slightly different perspective, psychoanalysts such as Sinason (1992) argue that frequent changes in terminology and policy shield us from acknowledging our discomfort with the realities of intellectual disability.

Clegg and Lansdall-Welfare (2003) conclude that concern to protect what little meaning people can create explains why many of those involved in intellectual disability services prefer simple ideas, and sometimes assert them dogmatically. A related perspective on the way people who are engaged with intellectual disability protect themselves comes from Gleeson (2003), who observed that intellectual disability services fall into unhelpfully simplistic "moral binaries". By this he refers to a range of simplistic ideas, such as "mainstream good, specialist bad" or "social good, medical bad". Such ideas conjure a two-dimensional world that is ill-equipped to comprehend the nuances of human experience. So, what research perspectives should be taken into account? One question is whether a "good" transition has been conceptualized appropriately when it focuses only on the young person. An important research theme concerns the difficulties carers face that are commonly ignored because carers have been "demoralized", their views and needs pushed beyond the moral pale (Gleeson, 2003). Hubert (1991) was one of the first researchers to describe such difficulties for carers of people with severe intellectual disabilities and challenging behaviour at the transition to adult services. Hanley-Maxwell, Whitney-Thomas, and Pogoloff (1995) identified high stress levels at this transition for all carers whose children have intellectual disabilities. The realization that their lives were going to diverge significantly from those of their peers started to sink home in what was described as "the second shock", encapsulating how many found this transition almost as shocking as the original diagnosis. Todd and Shearn (1997) described how carers also have to make a transition, to become parents of adults rather than children with intellectual disabilities. In another context, Pascall and Hendy (2004) showed that young people with physical disabilities who described their parents as "exceptional" fared best in terms of work and independence. Parents were crucial as carers, in developing independence, in mediating with professionals, and in providing material help to young people most likely to enter adulthood in poverty.

The well-being of other members of the system may also be relevant. On international comparison (Cummins, 2001), only in high-spending Sweden did parents of children with intellectual disabilities have similar levels of subjective well-being to parents of children without disabilities. Adaptability is one of the first resources that people lose when they struggle with everyday life, so limited carer flexibility could be a complementary explanation for difficult transitions.

* * *

The literature reviewed here provides a wealth of information about carer experiences with which practitioners could sensitize themselves. Such research is generally overlooked by PCP, which attends to the young person, not his or her network. To focus fully on the needs of every member of the system, and have new possibilities to keep at the back of their minds, systemic practitioners need to draw on all types and sources of information.

Expect engagement and disengagement

The final issue concerns people whose engagement with services is precarious. Typically, missed appointments at child and adolescent services in UK health services run at around 30%. Madsen (1999) describes how unhelpful, complementary relationships can then develop: worried services become intrusive, while multi-stressed families protect themselves from frequent intrusion through behaviour that invites the label "resistant". The more practitioners intrude, the more families resist. As soon as services employ the label resistant, they close down the space where they might envisage how life could be different, confining families to the life they have now. Elizur (1993) shows how recognizing unhelpful patterns between services and families is the first step towards more creative conversations. Successful ones open possibilities, conjuring different futures worth working for. Yet naïve optimism does people a disservice too, and it may equally result in them disengaging from services. Saetersdal (1997) described naivety in a different direction when she complained about the "Pollyanna" nature of intellectual disability services. Being too positive when people's lives or environments are grim makes it impossible for people to discuss real difficulties associated with the disabled life. Madsen (1999) suggests three guidelines for engaging multi-stressed people and families:

1. *Get to know them as people beyond the influence of their problems.* This provides connections that allow practitioners to sidestep problems of "resistance".
2. *Honour before helping.* Do not try to help until invited to do so. Until the invitation comes, focus on aspects of their lives that are working and admirable.
3. *Keep the problem on the table.* Once a problem they would like to work on has been identified, you are responsible for maintaining purpose. If there is continual drift away from the problem, renegotiate: do they no longer consider this the most important goal? Is there anything more important they would like to work on instead? People can take a while to identify what they will commit themselves to changing; others may have found the right problem to tackle, but not be used to seeing anything through. de Shazer (1988) invited practitioners to consider whether their clients were "visitors", "complainants", or "customers". This distinction is useful when addressing issues of engagement and saves unnecessary therapeutic effort. For visitors who do not have an identified problem they wish to address, de Shazer recommends acting as a good host: welcoming them and offering them compliments. Complainants come to complain about someone else whom they believe to be the problem. The practitioner's role is then to listen to them, and possibly to invite them to notice when the problem is less in evidence. Only customers agree that they have a problem and that you may have something to offer to help towards its solution. They are ready to engage in therapeutic work and can be given tasks that involve doing rather than merely observing.

Another way to address the issue of engagement is to consider the therapeutic alliance, considered crucial to the change process in all other psychotherapies. Wilson (1998b) describes with characteristic good humour how there is no single way to practice that will suit all clients. Some "chaotic" people want an authority figure they can have faith in to get them organized, others find that authoritative therapists fail to nurture their own change-creating resources. Some people want a poet whose playful engagement with words and metaphors makes discussion of painful matters possible, others are enraged by the poet's lack of clarity or direction. All that practitioners can do is introduce approaches that may be helpful, while checking how the clients experience them. Wilson encapsulates the therapist's role as follows: "To look for the contradictions in the descriptions people bring and to help open up new possibilities based on the child's, the parents' and the therapists' resourcefulness" (1998a, p. 2). Connecting with different needs and expectations, and keeping in mind different types of therapeutic alliance, can encourage the flexibility required to engage people who usually reject services. Persisting in environments that make rejection and failure common also needs good supervisory support.

Transition experiences and vignettes

Families with a person with intellectual disability often have life cycles that are unusual. For example, one or both parents may retire or become seriously ill just as the person leaves school or home. Such transitions may coincide with a sister leaving home and having her first baby. All parties may be affected: the person with intellectual disability may lose his or her main confidante while being reminded of a life-event they are unlikely to share; the sister may feel squeezed between expectations to create her own life while also "looking out for" her sibling; the mother may find her expectations of grandmotherhood compromised if her disabled child becomes jealous and attacks the new infant. Contemporary culture provides few life-narratives to inform such unusual coincidences, making them difficult to think or talk about.

In UK intellectual disability services, a fixed transition from child to adult services usually occurs at the age of 19 years, although for a few it occurs earlier, at 16 years. What Imber-Black (1988) describes as a service mandate does not necessarily synchronize with any change in the family's process: they may experience the transition as an arbitrary change that disrupts settled and satisfactory support arrangements. It forces them and their son or daughter to find a way through the contradictions of being described as an adult without meeting the ordinarily taken-for-granted criteria for adulthood. They may be most conscious of the loss of services and feel bewildered by the different expectations of new service systems. A common example of shifts at this transition is found in the different perspectives taken by child and adult staff employed by social services. While many staff in services for children usually prioritize helping parents to cope with their severely disabled son or daughter ("we never separate children from their families"), those in adult services are more likely to push for a move out of the family home ("she/he's an adult now, you need to learn to let go"). Indeed, some families complain that this is the only solution that community staff propose, whatever problem they may be experiencing.

* * *

Having no benchmarks about realistic expectations of change underpins many difficulties for people and their families. They are caught between unchanging organic aspects of the disability while wishing for development and "normal" transitions to take place. This may be amplified by workers in the service who can minimize disability. Complementary dynamics between families and staff can occur, one emphasizing hope for change, the other the unchanging nature of disability. When such complementarities are reflected in staff alliances with different family members, a polarized system results. Helping people to move from the hope that their idea will triumph to a situation where the system agrees on a shared direction of travel requires therapists, as they negotiate, to see a grain of truth in both positions.

The following vignettes illustrate some of the transition issues we have encountered, indicating briefly how we worked with the people and to what effect. We have deliberately omitted unnecessary detail and narrativized other components; the stories here illustrate our ideas—they are not comprehensive presentations.

Side-step autonomy

Joe, who has a mild level of intellectual disability, was referred for assessment when 19 years old. His parents were struggling to cope with his "oddness" and expressed a "desperate" wish for him to move out. A place was eventually found for him in a group home. He seemed to settle in well, and staff felt that he was "chilled out". However, his parents were very concerned, and they constantly telephoned the home with questions or complaints. An escalating complementarity developed: the more concerned and distressed the parents were at the perceived failure of the staff to take care of their son, the more group-home staff emphasized the positives to counter what they saw as the parents' refusal to let go. Only when Joe started to lose weight did some rapprochement became possible: there was no denying that he had some difficulties. It became clear that Joe had contributed to the complementarity by telling staff that everything was fine but expressing a great deal of anxiety to his parents at weekends, which they then fed back into the escalating pattern. During therapy we side-stepped invitations to arbitrate in the dispute between care and autonomy. Rather, we reflected the complementary pattern to both staff and parents. The suggestion arose of facilitating communication between parents and staff by channelling it through the manager, who was able to join with the views of both sides. We also worked in the clinic with the parental couple to help them with the transition.

* * *

Jane was a 21-year-old woman with mild intellectual disability in transition to adulthood. She lived within a close-knit system including a father, Tom, who had become mentally ill when Jane's older sister had moved out. Tensions in the current father–daughter relationship revolved largely around Jane's wish to enjoy the grown-up pleasures of alcohol and sex, while avoiding the move into independent adulthood that might disturb her beloved father's fragile emotional state again. Multiple losses and mutual protectionism gave a context to their difficulties, echoing Goldberg et al.'s (1995) experiences. The family did not find it possible to discuss loss with us until we had worked together for five months. This followed from a second exploration of family history, prompted by Tom repeatedly describing parenting as burdensome. When asked about the nature of that burden, Tom explained how he was compensating for neglect and abuse from his own father, and how his sister losing her child in an accident had made him more determined than ever to keep his children safe. He was enacting what Byng-Hall (1995) would describe as a reparative script. As we spoke, Tom said he realized for the first time how his older daughter had had to create a major row in order to leave home, otherwise he could not have let her go either. While at one level the matter was about the transition to adulthood, it needed to be approached by side-stepping the obvious letting-go discussion in favour of striving to understand

Tom's perspective. As he gained a metaperspective on himself which enabled a degree of psychological separation, Jane found it more possible to move into the world without his protection.

Keep multiple realities alive

The transition to adulthood can be a circuitous route navigated through abuse, loss of birth family, and settling into fostering. Researched extensively in services for children (Gorell Barnes, Thompson, Daniel, & Burchardt, 1998; Gorell Barnes & Dowling, 2000), such reconstituted or reordered family arrangements attract little attention in intellectual disability services.

* * *

Doris and Davina: Doris, a warm and experienced carer within an adult-placement scheme (a type of fostering), asked for support in her relationship with Davina, an 18-year-old with mild intellectual disability. Doris experienced Davina's self-harm as a "slap in the face". She knew Davina had been sexually and emotionally abused, but she could not comprehend why Davina continued to self-injure now she was in Doris's safe and accepting home. Angry arguments happened whenever Doris discovered further self-injury. This invited Davina to conceal; Doris could not bear such deceit but could not bear to discover the injuries either. Frustration at the discovery of significant further self-injury resulted in an argument that felt "like a bomb exploding in the household". The placement was close to breaking down.

There were two main strands to the work. We considered how Davina might let Doris know she had hurt herself, and get the support she needed, in a way that would be least upsetting to Doris. This was facilitated by Doris indicating that she hated the deceit more than the self-injury. She came to realize that her demands for Davina to promise it would never happen again gave deceit a stronger foothold. However, she continued to be mystified by the behaviour and pressed for advice about it. Following Fredman's (1997) recommendations that therapists should provide information as long as they have no investment in it being accepted, a one-page summary of general research findings about women who self-injure was provided at the next session, as a basis for discussing which aspects did and did not match her experience. This discussion allowed Davina to discuss the urge to hurt herself with Doris for the first time. Davina developed an analogy between her self-injury and drinkers in Alcoholics Anonymous, facilitating discussion of how survivors get on with life while accepting that occasional relapses are likely. After four sessions, Doris said nothing much had changed, except that Davina's self-harming had got less severe and less frequent and that she herself became less upset and responded differently when it happened. The therapeutic task had been helping them to find their own ways to understand and respond to self-injury. In part this appeared to be learning how to live with, rather than deny, the history of abuse that had entered the household. They ceased attending the clinic, with continuing support provided to Davina individually. One year later, Davina sent a message to the clinic that she had not hurt herself for the previous twelve months and that her brother had been arrested for sexually abusing children, and she had testified against him, without recurrence of self-harm.

Expect engagement and disengagement

As change proceeds slowly in intellectual disability services, and as families remain in the service even when they stop attending the clinic (permanently or temporarily), the point at which to evaluate outcome is ambiguous.

* * *

Charlie: The parents of Charlie (aged 20, mild intellectual disability) attended sessions for close to eighteen months concerning his violence, especially towards his mother. There was great ambivalence on the part of all family members regarding the possibility of Charlie moving out of the family home. They terminated family therapy, stating that it was not really helping. Charlie himself said that he found the family meetings too painful. He continued in individual therapy, and social-work input continued to the family. Five years after the start of family therapy, and three years after its end, he moved to his own flat. Retrospectively, all involved felt that the family therapy had laid the foundations for this change, together with systemically informed individual therapy and a systemic approach to the review meetings. Had outcome been measured at the end of clinic attendance, this would not have been noted.

* * *

Pamela: A family with a daughter Pamela (30 years old, with severe intellectual disability) displayed a pattern of contact with the clinic that had recurred in their contact with all services. They would attend appointments or be in for home visits once or twice, apparently engaged, only to drop from contact. There were clear and strong emotions between all family members, whose concern was most easily expressed by becoming angry and frustrated with one another. Pamela became distressed during one session, her mother cried during another, and we suspect that becoming overwhelmed made it difficult for them all to continue. They were clearly not coping together but lacked the resources to change their relationships; the parents were also reluctant to entrust Pamela to services they had not found trustworthy. During therapy we held a "when-or-if" discussion ("Are we talking about *when* you decide or *if* you decide that Pamela should go into residential care?"): they agreed "when" as the general frame, but both parents differed about how soon "when" should come. Pamela's mother continued to place hunting for the perfect home above meeting their needs as a couple; her father was at his most engaged when expressing his hopes for a companionable retirement before they became too old to enjoy it. They ceased to attend therapy, but a month later their community worker asked us to offer them another appointment. We suggested a three-way appointment, so that the worker could offer them support and we could review together why she thought it would be helpful for them to return. The parents agreed to the proposal but did not attend, although the worker did. We discussed how we might understand their intermittent contact with services, and we wrote them a brief therapeutic letter summarizing our thinking. Therapeutic letters (White & Epston, 1990) are generally a move within an ongoing therapeutic relationship, but they can also be used to communicate concern to people for whom the engagement is precarious. This summarized the "when-or-if" conversation of previous sessions and signalled our concern for them. We heard later that the parents had cited this letter as significant in prompting them to seek a community placement for Pamela more actively and to face the difficulties that moving out would entail. Unfortunately, that worker left three months later, before a placement had been identified. The pattern of engagement–disengagement with services continues.

***

Simon: Another family attended with concerns about the behaviour of Simon (age 17 years, with a mild intellectual disability). Relationships between him, his mother, and his stepfather were fraught, culminating in regular angry outbursts by Simon. After six sessions, there were many stories of positive developments in Simon and in family togetherness. His 18th birthday was being anticipated as a significant ritual marking a passage to a new stage. Therapy was therefore terminated. Within the next few months the mother made contact with three different professionals about concerns regarding Simon. These people were sufficiently systemically informed to question the need for individually focused work. Eventually the mother contacted the clinic again, six months after the end of the previous intervention. She and her husband attended for some sessions to address their differences of approach in managing Simon as well as the effect of those differences on their relationship and on the family atmosphere. The mother felt that her relatively new husband was too confrontational with Simon; he could not bear to see his wife insulted by her son. A dialogue was possible around the relative effectiveness of different approaches on Simon's responses. Once again the situation was described as greatly improved. Depending on how or where we had punctuated the work with this family, we might have described the "outcome" as successful or unsuccessful.

* * *

Our thinking about families' engagement with service systems enabled us to raise explicitly with these parents the question of the repeating pattern of engagement and disengagement. We noted that they had twice attended in the autumn with problems, then felt that things were better in the late spring. We addressed possible reasons for this pattern, with a view to preventing a repeat the following year.

Conclusions

We side-step the frequent push within services to promote autonomy in order to see more clearly the interdependencies that are so crucial to systemic thinking. Joe illustrated how need for care has to be balanced against need for autonomy; Jane showed the importance of understanding her father's narratives and their family history before it was possible to comprehend their difficulty in separating from each other.

Research can alert us to ideas that may be important but missing; conceptual analyses suggest why the discursive world of intellectual disability tends to prefer simple ideas. Both create a space where multiple narratives can coexist. Davina's story illustrates how providing expert information when a system requests it can be compatible with postmodern practice if it expands the clients' range of understanding while leaving them to interpret and apply it.

Finally, we explored difficulties with therapeutic engagement from a variety of research and practice orientations. Many clients, families, and systems face multiple problems that make it likely that their engagement with services will be ambivalent at best. Working relationships that were difficult to create are inevitably disrupted by frequent service change as well as transitions. Charlie, Pamela, and Simon provide different perspectives on how practitioners may understand and work with families whose contact with services is intermittent.

Current policies on transition offer little succour to families with complex needs. It is unlikely that more experience of change, and smoother service coordination, will resolve their difficulties. For people who are only just coping, transitions bring huge challenges. Our task is to be alongside people, enabling them to develop and act on realistic hopes, by reflecting, negotiating, and renegotiating.

Reflections

Jennifer Clegg
It has been a real pleasure to reflect both on the various ways that systemic ideas have excited and refreshed my practice and also to appreciate colleagues and clients who were willing to try doing things differently. Holding onto multiple realities that include ideas I find uncongenial is one of the central challenges of systemic work for me: family therapy training has made it more likely I can stop to ask myself what is happening when I feel strong antipathy towards an idea. Why has my ability to appreciate the other perspective become so sharply narrowed? Is it the people, the topic, the context? I suspect that risk is a great narrower of perspectives, and demeaning talk of all kinds, but probably I am also challenged when things get more complicated than I can manage. In services where review meetings occasionally run on for hours, discursive chaos is a realistic fear.

Susan King
I also notice that I am least tolerant of a "reality" (see, I have to put it in quotes) that does not support the concept of multiple realities. I am

certain that certainty is a bad thing—and I am particularly intolerant when I see intolerance in people who I feel "should know better", usually experienced staff members. Those situations are the ones in which supervision and opportunities to reflect are invaluable. It is useful to be reminded that thinking in uncertainty and multiplicity is strange for many. I also need to recall that there are times when multiplicity is not useful. I need to curb my knee-jerk tendency to open up more and more possibilities, and to remember the usefulness of focus. As has been said: "We do not want to be so open-minded that our brains fall out."

CHAPTER EIGHT

Who needs to change? Using systemic ideas when working in group homes

Selma Rikberg Smyly

Why systemic?

"Experience is not what happens to you. It is what you do with what happens to you."

Aldous Huxley (1932, p. 5)

My intention in this chapter is to give you an idea of why I became interested in systemic ideas and to outline some of the theoretical concepts that have been particularly important in influencing my thinking. I also demonstrate through two examples, which describe in more detail the connections between theory and practice, how I have used these ideas when working in group homes.

* * *

What makes ideas appeal to us? Is it their innate complexity and elegance, or is it the manner in which a point of view can be convincingly and well argued? Maybe it is the empirical evidence of effectiveness, which draws us to a particular theory? Maybe—but maybe it is also an inner resonance with particular ideas, as if one had heard it somewhere before, as if in the recesses of our memory lurked some half-forgotten ideas that suddenly become focused. This sense of familiarity, recognition, and instant appeal is likely to have as much to do with our personal histories and experiences as it has with the theories themselves. A typical systemic answer to the above questions would, in fact, be "both . . . and". What one often forgets, though, is the personal aspect of this appeal, and what one might perhaps emphasize is the quality, usefulness, or evidence base of the theories themselves.

* * *

When, as a clinical psychologist, I was taking part in systemic/family therapy training at the Oxford Family Institute, I was curious about the systemic articles we read and how different they were to many clinical psychology publications. One of the differences I appreciated was the way in which the authors tended to be explicit about their theoretical biases and personal focus of interests. In fact, they offered readers the opportunity to position themselves in relation to the article and in relation to the authors. Emphasizing the fact that this was one "story" written from one particular perspective made it clearer and easier to evaluate its relevance in relation to other articles and other theoretical perspectives.

* * *

So, why am I interested in systemic ideas, and what does it mean to me? In a sense, it was a "home-coming" experience for me. Listening to the lectures and workshops, I became aware that these were indeed not new ideas; social constructionism was familiar to me from my early days as an undergraduate studying at Birmingham University for a joint honours degree in sociology and psychology. I particularly enjoyed anthropology, which had probably something to do with the fact that I was brought up in a bilingual and bi-cultural home in Finland. After I trained in the UK, I worked for five years in Zimbabwe, and it was here that I was first introduced to Milan-based family therapy. Its cultural sensitivity and relevance impressed me at a time when I was struggling to find culturally acceptable ways of applying psychological theory in such a different setting. For me, it became clear that in order to understand what is taking place around us—for example, someone's behaviour—we need to understand the attitudes and beliefs that inform these behaviours. Attitudes and beliefs are influenced by, and are deeply embedded in, the personal, familial, cultural, and social contexts we find ourselves in. "Meaning making" of our lives is as much of a social process as it is a personal one (Hannah, 1994). Having been fortunate enough to live in a number of different cultural contexts and being used to hearing, seeing, and living alternative explanations about the same life events, my personal life experiences confirmed the basic ideas of a socially constructed reality. It is, therefore, perhaps not so surprising that I have found myself particularly drawn to social constructionist and narrative ideas and that these ideas are increasingly beginning to inform my practice.

* * *

Working as a clinical psychologist in an intellectual disabilities context, I was struck by the sense of powerlessness in the lives of our clients. If our lives are seen as storied within the social contexts we live in (White & Epston, 1990), then for this client group the reality was often that they were storied *for* them. How could the frequently problem-saturated dominant stories be changed into more positive and inclusive stories of the multiple views and perspectives held by the people involved? In particular, how could the emphasis change from predominantly professional descriptions of clients to the views of the carer, the family, and, most importantly, the client about what was happening? How could all of the different stories be seen to make sense or even be heard? I found my role in this to be one of meaning making, of finding and encouraging alternative or subjugated stories, and, by encouraging more inclusive conversations, allowing new stories to emerge.

* * *

The theoretical ideas that I found particularly helpful come from the social constructionist perspective developed by people like Andersen (1987, 1991), Anderson and Goolishian (1988, 1992), Boscolo and Bertrando (1996), Cecchin (1992), Cecchin, Lane, and Ray (1992), Cronen (1994), Hoffman (1990, 1993), McNamee and Gergen (1992). Some of these ideas have been excellently summarized more recently by Ekdawi et al. (2000).

* * *

From these ideas I found the important shift in thinking involving the move from first- to second-order cybernetics particularly interesting. This was initially described by Howe and von Foerster (1974) and formed the basis for questioning the position of the practitioner as a neutral, objective outsider to the family system (first-order cybernetics). Instead, the practitioner became seen as being influenced by the system as well as influencing it. In fact, patterns of mutual influence develop (second-order cybernetics). As Anderson and Goolishian (1992, p. 27) point out, "The therapist becomes the participant observer and participant facilitator of the therapeutic conversation". As a result, therapy became seen as a process whereby we mutually co-create or re-author new stories and meanings together with the relevant people concerned through the dynamic process of conversation (White & Epston, 1990; White, 1991). Conceptually this is achieved not from a position of the "outside expert", but from an acknowledgement of subjectivity on each side. This position as expounded by these authors, among others, has become known as the "not-knowing position" or the "non-expert" model of working. From this position of a "participant observer", our views and expertise are merely another possible story/description to explain what might be happening, which, together with all the alternative views offered by other participants, inform the process of finding the most helpful stories. These are the stories that help to make most sense to the system or the family of the current situation and offer the most opportunities for moving forward. "There are no truths, only more or less helpful ways of seeing a problem" (Gergen, 1994, p. 33).

* * *

Another influential shift in thinking involved the focus in social constructionist ideas on meanings and attitudes, as opposed to actual behaviours or events. For social constructionists, truths or events are not discovered but constructed. It is the underlying beliefs about a situation that inform our point of view or action. Therapeutically the uncovering or deconstructing of these beliefs in conversation is seen as a central focus of the conversation (Hoffman, 1990). By widening the context of the conversations (Cronen, 1994) and including as many relevant family and network points of view, the meanings and beliefs underlying actions can more easily be discerned and the possibility of alternative stories and possible new actions created. In order for new meanings and stories to emerge, I have found using different ways of applying reflecting-team conversations a particularly helpful method for introducing "news of difference" (Bateson, 1972). Tom Andersen's work on reflecting teams has been particularly influential (Andersen, 1987, 1991, 1995). In my work context, working as part of a multidisciplinary team for an NHS Trust, we do not have the luxury of one-way screens with video facilities. More often than not the "reflecting team"—usually one or possibly two colleagues—sit in the session with a staff group or client. However, by adapting the use of reflecting teams, as Andersen demonstrates, one can use the therapeutic intent of reflecting teams by introducing certain adaptations. For example, when working with staff teams, I often use part of the staff team as a reflecting team while the other half discusses an issue. Or I may interview one staff member while others are asked to first listen and then discuss together their thoughts about the interview. I have also interviewed the referred client with two staff-team members present, who listen and then reflect on the conversation. Or the other way round: two members of staff have a conversation, which I have then reflected on with the referred client. In this sense, some of these conversations become closer to what Michael White describes as outsider-witness groups (White, 1999), in that they involve groups of people who are not practitioners themselves. However, some of the key features of giving clients, carers, and practitioners an opportunity to hear how what is being said is being heard, understood, or interpreted by others—and how this enables stories to be elaborated on, with new information being introduced—remain central.

Why are systemic ideas helpful in group homes?

> "In therapy, we listen to a story and then we collaborate with the person we are seeing to invent other stories or other meanings for the stories that are told."
>
> Hoffman (1990, p. 11).

In this section I briefly describe why I became interested in applying systemic ideas to my work with staff groups; I and then outline some of the key features of these ideas before presenting two examples from my practice to illustrate more practically this way of working.

* * *

Within different service settings, different challenges become apparent. For me it was the referrals from staffed group homes. In my experience, these particular settings were often not receptive to traditional psychological interventions and remained often uninfluenced and probably unimpressed by them. Many multidisciplinary-team colleagues felt that despite spending a lot of time trying to explain our point of view about a client's problem and the possible solutions to staff teams, nothing seemed to change.

* * *

I felt that the systemic stance of working from a non-expert position, trying not to prescribe solutions, seemed particularly pertinent to these settings. These complex systems operated somewhat like families where carers varyingly defined their roles as friends, advocates, supporters of independent lifestyles, and so on and were unarguably "experts" on the clients. Who were we in the team, coming from the outside, to tell anybody what they should do? With our limited knowledge of clients or the realities involved in running a group home, we were ill-equipped to provide "expert opinions". One of the key issues for me became, therefore, how we merge these multiple perspectives—the different bits of expert knowledge provided variously by carers, clients, family members, and professionals involved—to make a story that made sense to the whole system and enabled people to move on and create new situations, new actions, and new stories about the clients as well as themselves.

Systemic ideas applied to organizational settings

From the literature on working systemically in organizations, I have found the writings by Campbell, Coldicott, and Kinsella (1994), Huffington and Brunning (1994), and Campbell (2000) helpful in outlining possible models that seem particularly relevant. These incorporate many of the central ideas within a second-order cybernetics and social constructionist frame of systemic thinking (e.g., the FORSEE approach in Campbell, Coldicott, & Kinsella, 1994, pp. 123–147). They provide many helpful pointers to working in organizational settings, and the following is my adaptation of some of these ideas for working in group homes. In this work with group homes, I have found three key areas important to consider. These include what I call the agency life-cycle stage; beliefs, attitudes, and expectations of the staff team; and, probably most importantly, methods used to engage in conversation with the staff team.

Agency life-cycle stage

Organizationally speaking, any "system" will encounter challenges at times of change—hence the need to consider the current situation of the referring agency. For example, new clients moving into a group home, staff leaving, or newly established homes where structures and support networks have not yet been clarified are all potentially more challenging situations both for staff and clients and are hence more likely to generate referrals for the multidisciplinary team. At the initial referral from a group home, it is therefore often helpful to consider questions such as:

- Why is this referral being made now?
- For whom is the current referral issue a problem?
- How new or experienced is the staff group or agency?
- Is the client known or unknown to the staff group (i.e., recently moved in, or long-term resident)?

Other important considerations are the ethos of the organization and the roles staff are expected to assume. If the ethos is primarily about supporting people to be independent and a client begins to show signs of dementia, the staff roles and expectations may need to be re-evaluated. Other issues to consider are: Who should the practitioner work with? How will senior managers, parents, and other agencies view this referral? Who are the customers, in other words, who may have a vested interest in introducing change? What effect will these changes have on the staff and clients of the group home? Deeply divisive staff teams, where problems of recruitment, retention, or disciplinary issues arise, may need careful negotiation about how and with whom to engage. Often it is helpful to include senior managers and other relevant stakeholders in these initial conversations.

Beliefs, attitudes, and expectations of the staff team

Considering staff, family, and professional views about the presenting problem, and, in particular, what beliefs might inform these views, is an important beginning. As Reder and Fredman (1996) have pointed out, the expectations about the input offered may vary depending on, for example, previous experience of help. It is therefore helpful at this stage not only to identify those who comprise the relevant network, but also to find out what their connection to and perception of the referred problem might be.

- What beliefs are there about the client's current problems and behaviours?
- What beliefs are there about the client's disability and how this may effect the client?
- What knowledge is there of life history and of contact with family and friends?
- What differences of beliefs are there between different agencies, carers working with the client, and the client themselves?
- What is the history of the problem and solutions attempted?
- What part did outside agencies, such as the multidisciplinary team, play previously, and what might therefore be the expectations now?
- What was seen as particularly helpful or not helpful in the past?

These are questions that seek to place the problem in context. In addition, it is the beginnings of trying to create meanings around the behaviour, to provide a broader base of ideas from which new information may emerge. It also establishes who are part of the relevant network and who may need to be involved in the work.

Encouraging participative conversations

It is important to consider how answers to the above questions are sought and who needs to be part of this process. As mentioned above, ideally this needs to be considered and agreed on from the beginning. The most helpful way of doing this may vary at different times and in different contexts, but as a rule of thumb it is helpful to try to involve as many relevant people from the network of concern as possible. In intellectual disability services, the challenge is often about the involvement of the client in this process and how to find helpful and supportive ways of doing so. In my experience, the least helpful way is for the outside agency—in this case, members of the multidisciplinary team—to engage with only one person from the staff team without actively seeking the views and ideas from the rest of the staff team/family and client. If only one dominant view is sought, the result is often just a repeat of the "problem-saturated story", and the opportunity to hear alternative stories is diminished. Neither is it helpful to take the "outside-expert" role and interview a whole network of people individually. When working in this way, I often felt overburdened by the sheer volume of different stories, frequently contradicting each other, and found it hard to come up with diplomatic ways of sharing this information with the relevant network. Being the information gatherer and holder is being in a position of power. One is then in a position to decide which bits of information to share and what actions to take. However, this way of operating from an "expert model" has both limited usefulness and all the possible frustrations described earlier.

* * *

A systemic approach offers the opportunity of a potentially more participative way of engaging the "network" in sharing stories/information and enabling the network to make sense of what these stories may mean and, ultimately, what may need to change to help the client. Beliefs/attitudes/descriptions held by the different parts of the network need to be heard and reflected on by the people involved. The relevance of this information is determined by the feedback the system gives and the sense it makes of what this shared information means. It also helps in avoiding putting the practitioner in the assumed role of the expert who has come to "fix" the problem. As pointed out by Cecchin and his colleagues: "be careful, because if therapists give the illusion that they can do something, then the system will buy the illusion of power" (Cecchin, Lane, & Ray, 1992, p. 6).

First example

In this and the next example from my work, my aim is to demonstrate in practice some of the approaches outlined in the preceding section.

Working in a group home: John's story

A referral was made to the multidisciplinary team (MDT) I work in from a manager of a small group home with three residents. This group home catered for clients with more moderate to severe intellectual disabilities. The referral concerned the challenging behaviour of one of the male residents, John (aged 55) who was described as "occasionally physically violent towards staff members". The referral was allocated to me as the psychologist on the team. A nurse from the team had already been working with the client.

Agency "life-cycle stage"

From a telephone conversation I had with the manager who made the referral, it transpired that she was new to the group home and had made the referral after observing some of John's challenging behaviour. The current staff team had experienced a number of changes in the past year, with three staff leaving (out of a total of nine). This had resulted in agency staff being used on a fairly regular basis. The client was targeting some members of the staff team, and this had caused some friction in the team. These particular issues had a long history and a number of referrals had been made to the MDT over the years. This staff group also supported another house next-door, with two further clients living in it.

At this early stage I find it helpful to set the context for the work (e.g., who are the members of the relevant network, and who should be at an initial meeting to discuss the referral). I tend to be guided by the referrer in deciding who needs to come to initial meetings, ensuring that I offer the option of all relevant people in the network to attend. In such initial meetings it is helpful for the practitioner to keep in mind those not present and to frequently check with the people involved who else may need to be part of these conversations and how to gradually include these others in this process. In this particular situation, we agreed on an initial meeting that included the whole staff team and the community nurse. The client, however, was not included at this stage, as he was unaware of the referral.

Engaging staff teams in conversations

The information I had gained from the initial telephone call with the referrer helped me to plan the first session. A number of issues struck me about the above conversation, which prompted some initial hypotheses about what might be going on in this group home. There were staff in the group home who had known John a long time, and there were also those who had left, with stories about John that may have been lost. In addition there were new staff members, including the manager, who were, in a sense, trying to "find their feet". How had John experienced these changes? How did the staff team view these changes? How, if at all, did this relate to the referral problem? What, if anything, had helped in the past? I was particularly interested in knowing if staff who had known John for a long time had different views about the above issues from those staff members who had only recently arrived. I saw the aim of the first session as creating a context within which the views of as many participants as possible could be heard in a supportive and respectful way. My role would be specifically to enable and facilitate such conversations to take place. The aim would be to broaden the perceptions of the referred problem by looking at, and sharing, alternative explanations and beliefs about the perceived problem and, in this way, create a context for new and different conversations to take place about what was happening for John.

Using reflecting conversations in group homes

Since I use reflecting conversations in a relatively broad manner, as mentioned earlier, I do not tend to give lengthy explanations about the theory or about my systemic orientation at this stage. As a way of explanation I might say something like, "People often have different views about what is going on, and I have found it important to give everyone in the room an opportunity to speak as well as listen. Doing this in a more structured way can sometimes be helpful." I always offer the initial session as an experiment, which we do not need to repeat if it proves to be unhelpful.

* * *

In this initial staff meeting, I asked the participants to group themselves into four pairs in such a way that each pair consisted of someone relatively new to working with John and someone who had known him for a longer time. From my hypothesizing and the brief discussion we had before the reflecting conversation, I expected and observed staff to have different views about John depending on how long they had worked in the house. In order to ensure that these views and differences were given an opportunity to be heard, staff who may not always work together or share the same views were chosen to work in pairs. These pairs were asked to consider the following two questions: "Why do you think John becomes upset?" "What have you found helpful in the past when he has been upset?"

This was followed by me interviewing one of the pairs about their conversation, clarifying the points they were making, highlighting differences and similarities in their views, and, if necessary, asking for further information. Prior to doing this, I asked the three other pairs to listen to my interview of the first pair, bearing the following two questions in mind: "How similar or different was their conversation about John to the one they were hearing?" "What, if anything, surprised them about what they heard?"

Following the initial interview of the first pair, I asked the three other pairs to share, in turn, their response to what they had heard. In this manner, we gradually built a number of stories about the reasons for John's apparent upset and how best to help him. Each pair contributed their unique conversation and highlighted the aspects of their story that were similar to or different from what they had heard when listening to the interview.

Themes from staff "reflecting conversations": beliefs, attitudes, and expectations

Three main themes emerged from the above conversations. First, John had apparently always singled out the newest members of staff for his "attacks". People felt that this was possibly due to his feeling uncomfortable or worried with new members of staff. Second, quite a clear difference emerged between those staff members who "did everything or most things" for John and those who felt that their role was to promote independence and therefore John's ability to "do things for himself". This view had split the staff-team members, with some antagonism shown by people holding opposite views. Third, apparently John found it difficult when staff left the house. Staff-team members were often suddenly called to go next-door to support the clients there. Staff leaving the house had for a long time been a potentially challenging situation, with John showing increasing signs of distress as people prepared to leave the house.

New emerging stories about John

When sharing these themes from the reflecting conversations with the staff team, a number of issues were clearly "new information" for some of the staff involved. For example, the newest member of staff no longer felt incompetent, because others had experienced what she was experiencing. The different staff views on how to support John was "new information" to the manager and other staff-team members and had not been expressed so clearly before. The disruption caused by having to cover two houses had been a long-term concern for the staff team and was an issue that the manager had felt strongly was not to the advantage of either house. The fact that this seemed to be a particularly stressful situation for John was highlighted.

* * *

Systemically, the opportunity to reframe some of the above themes was possible. For example, how to support John was not necessarily a matter of choosing one way over another. Both methods may be appropriate in different circumstances. From the staff stories, it was clear that there were times when doing things for John was important to make him feel cared for and that there were other times when encouraging him to do things for himself could make him feel more confident about himself. However, finding out when to adopt which approach was a priority. What could John's views be on this? It was suggested by the staff team that two staff members who had good relationships with John would, together with the community nurse, who had known him for many years, initiate conversations with John about this and explore his views. In fact this became part of his person-centred planning (PCP: Department of Health, 2002), an approach used by the organization to ensure individual participation in life planning which facilitated an ongoing conversation about helpful ways of supporting him in different situations.

* * *

The issue about why John was distressed when people left the house prompted a discussion about the potential confusion between people leaving to go home after a shift, leaving to go on holiday, or leaving to go to another job. This led to the question as to how the staff team could make their comings and goings less confusing for clients. The merits of "leaving rituals/parties" were discussed, as well as the possibility of photographs of who was on duty that day, with separate pictures of those on holiday/off sick, and so forth. The question of the stresses involved in supporting two different houses led to the agreed preference of splitting into two smaller staff teams, with separate support provided for each house.

Outcomes

The above session was the only staff meeting I was involved with. The only additional input was a further telephone conversation with the home manager six weeks later. From this conversation it transpired that the PCP process had helped to make John's views about how he wanted to be supported central to how the staff team saw their roles (i.e., caring versus supporting independence) and enabled the conflict between staff to become less of an issue. The staff team had also initiated putting photographs of people on duty in a prominent place and, in a separate place, photographs of those who had left. Another change had been achieved in that the staff team, with management support, was now beginning to operate as two separate teams in the two houses, with far fewer overlaps. Moreover, there had been a clear reduction in the number of incidents of aggressive behaviour. When they had occurred, the staff team was clearer about the reason for this and felt able to make necessary changes to improve the situation. For example, staff were more aware of how they left the house, giving more information to John about why they were leaving and when they were due to be back.

* * *

From a systemic point of view, my role had been to facilitate conversations about John in such a way that the staff team shared with each other new explanations and information about possible alternative meanings to the problem and hence were able to find alternative ways of solving the problem. Even though John had not joined this initial conversation, his role became increasingly central in informing the staff team, through the PCP process, about his preferred ways of support. John's voice became gradually more influential in his own life and, as a consequence, the "stories" about him less negative and more balanced.

Reflections on the work

The above example was an attempt at working from a non-expert position together with a staff team. My position as the facilitator left me with no clear role in the subsequent work with the client. Previously I would have volunteered to "do" much of the needed legwork—for example, going to talk to other members of the network not present at the meeting, such as a day-service provider, client, or family member, or becoming involved in the PCP process. However, it gradually dawned on me that this was not always useful. From my past experience, the practitioner knowing what others thought about the situation often made little difference. It was more likely to make a difference if members of the relevant system/network had access to this information and were able to reflect on it. In this particular example, I was also aware that not being involved in doing something left me in a position of little or no control. This felt inherently uncomfortable—I felt neither important nor needed! My position had shifted, I was no longer the outside expert who had come to "fix" the problem, but "merely" someone who had had a relatively useful conversation with a group of staff and a community nurse who subsequently got on with doing their jobs. It reminded me of a quote from Fruggeri (1992) describing therapy as the art of engaging in "a conversation, that particular kind of conversation that changes all the other conversations" (p. 49). However, maybe most importantly, I had changed my position in the system in such a way that other participants had an opportunity to contribute and become part of the "problem solvers".

Second example

I have included this second example to demonstrate the many and varied ways in which working systemically can take place. Unlike the above example, this work took approximately six months and consisted of a number of different conversations with different parts of the network of concern.

Working in group homes: Sue's story

Sue, who was 42 years of age, was referred to the MDT by her group-home manager. She was one of three residents in a group home that catered for people with mild intellectual disabilities with a high level of independent functioning. The referrer described a variety of difficult behaviours, not just at home but also at the day service. In addition, there were differences of opinion between her parents' views about how to deal with Sue and the staff's views about this.

Context of work

The context of this referral involved three linked but separate networks, all of which the client was a member of: the group home, the day service, and the family. Since the referral had come from only one of the parties concerned, the views about this referral needed to be clarified from the day-service, client, and parents' point of view. How were the issues above viewed by the other parts of the network, who else may be concerned, and who were our customers? Because I was, at the time, working with a colleague who was a trainee clinical psychologist particularly interested in systemic practice, this offered an opportunity to use reflecting conversations by using the trainee psychologist as my reflecting "team". Thus, unlike the previous example, I had the luxury of a co-worker.

Due to the conflicting views expressed by the referrer between the carers and parents, we decided to arrange a number of separate initial meetings with the different members of the network—that is, group-home and day-service staff; the client, together with her keyworker from the day service (client's choice); as well as the parents. This was to ensure that all different views could be heard, expressed, and respected without some stories predominating at the meeting. These preliminary meetings all followed a similar format: my colleague or I would interview the relevant network member(s), and halfway through this conversation we offered a reflection of what we had heard; following this, our reflections were commented on by the original contributors.

Using this process with someone who has intellectual disabilities raised some initial concerns about the client's willingness to contradict us if we got things wrong. Would our views and interpretations become the dominant ones? However, when working with Sue we were reassured on this issue by the many times she would say "No, you got that wrong", "It's not like that", and so forth when commenting on our reflections. By trying to make our thinking as transparent as possible, the process of reflecting on each other's point of view provided an opportunity to validate our stories and clarify our perceptions and assumptions about what was going on for Sue. It also offered an opportunity to explore ideas that Sue may have had difficulty expressing but was able to comment on if put into words with alternatives provided. For example, Sue at one point said that she wanted to "feel important" in her life but had found it difficult to put into words what she meant.

In our reflections to her, we discussed what this concept might mean to her and the times in her life when she might have felt important. By hearing us discuss several alternatives, she was able to pick out the ones that were relevant to her as well as add other ones we had not thought of. Working in this way provided us with a safeguard for getting the "story" right, exploring alternatives we may not have thought of, and widening the context of the initial conversation.

Themes emerging from our reflecting conversations: beliefs, attitudes, and expectations

In our sessions with Sue, a strong theme emerged of her own sense of confusion about her role in the group home as well as at the day service. Sue told us she was a "staff helper" and that her job was to help other clients. Since moving away from the family home, her options and choices seemed more limited. She had consistently chosen not to take part in activities. Yet she longed to feel "important" in her life. Some of the ways that made her feel important included participating in meetings and teaching skills to others. At the group home, Sue was seen as "bossy"—a person who did not like being told what to do and who often took the role of the decision-maker for others in the home. This had led to conflict between residents in the house as well as the staff team. Staff attempts at supporting Sue to become independent and make choices for herself were perceived as being undermined by her parents, who were seen to continue to make all decisions for her. This left staff feeling frustrated, undermined, and criticized by the parents.

* * *

Day-service staff described Sue as difficult to engage. When offered activities, she would always initially say "Yes" but then drop out. Sue wanted to join staff meetings at the day service and generally enjoyed organizing and being in meetings. However, this could sometimes be very intrusive, and she had to be reminded that staff meetings were not generally open for clients to attend.

Sue's parents described a lifelong dedication to providing the best possible care for their daughter. Sue had been taught many skills by the family, including cooking, crafts, and music, and the parents felt that Sue was currently losing these skills. Sue had always had a very clear role of helping at the family home, where she was referred to as "Mum's helper".

Moving to independent living involved a real sense of concern and confusion about what the parental role should be. How could one let go if staff appeared not to "care" for her appropriately? The parents had had some unfortunate experiences and misunderstandings with the residential staff and, as a consequence, felt that the staff did not understand their daughter.

The parents also described their sense of needing to protect their daughter by, for example, covering up her failings. Since other people could not possibly be as tolerant and understanding about Sue, it became important to make Sue appear as acceptable as possible. This entailed, among other things, telling her what to wear, as well as the need to point out "mistakes" she made when in the presence of other people.

Network meetings: encouraging participative conversations

Following our sessions with Sue, with the staff team, and with Sue's parents, a couple of combined network meetings were arranged. These meetings included all parties concerned except Sue. She seemed very content for us to "tell Mum and Dad" and not to be in the meeting herself. If the client is not going to be part of such meetings, I usually discuss with them what they would like me to share about our conversations.

In Sue's situation, discussing what made her feel important seemed central. Her sense of confusion seemed a very clear response to the changes in her life situation. By moving away from home, she seemed to have become a less, rather than more, important person. The transition from home to group home entailed a whole set of new roles for everyone concerned. However, somehow the negotiation of these new roles seemed not to have taken place. The conflicting expectations of Sue in the different settings added to her sense of confusion, and we therefore felt that prioritizing Sue's perspective of what was happening needed to be the central focus of the meeting. With Sue's agreement, we decided to present what we understood to be "Sue's story" to the meeting and asked the participants to discuss how well this represented their understanding of Sue. The story we presented focused on our perception of Sue's apparent confusion about her role and areas of control in her life; how she needed to feel "important"; and how each of us might help her with these issues.

* * *

Using the reflecting-team model, the group was divided into two smaller ones to consider our version of Sue's story. Each of these groups consisted of a day-service and group-home staff member and one parent. This was relatively easy to do as each part of the network was accustomed to our reflective format from our initial conversations with them. We asked the two groups to consider the following questions: "How well did our representation of Sue's point of view fit with their view of what was happening?" "Which explanations did we need to add or take away from this description?" Each group took turns in talking about their view about our representation of what was happening for Sue, followed by listening to and reflecting on the other group's conversation. Two particular issues were highlighted: first, the differences between how things used to be done at home with the family and how they were done now, and the way in which this was adding to Sue's sense of confusion; second, the fact that meetings about Sue were usually problem-focused. Suggestions were made for how this could change. This in turn raised the question of what changing from being "Mum's helper" to becoming a "staff helper" would involve.

One of the potentially influential conversations that we had involved a discussion between parents and the group-home staff about the differences in expectations between the two settings. We provided a forum for normalizing some of the problems in terms of general issues about leaving home as well as refocusing the tensions between the two settings in terms of the sense of confusion it caused for Sue.

Not uncommonly, in their endeavours to provide independent lifestyles where client choice is seen as central, group-home staff find themselves in direct opposition to parents who have for years fostered a much more nurturing and caring role with their son or daughter. Understanding that rules may be different in different places, that one is being allowed to make decisions in one place and have them made for one in another, are complex and often confusing experiences. Helping Sue and the relevant network make sense of these experiences therefore seemed very important.

Outcomes

Following these network meetings, Sue's role changed to being in charge of her own meetings and deciding who should attend them and what the agenda items were. The significant people in her life were helping her to define her role and legitimate areas of control and, in the process of doing so, were helping Sue to regain a sense of importance in her life.

From a systemic point of view, what had changed were the perceptions of why this person was being "difficult" and not fitting in. The stories told about Sue were no longer problem-saturated but included words such as "confused" and "needing more confidence". Bringing in Sue's story, even if second-hand, enabled new information and a different perspective to be considered. Exploring why people felt the need to do what they had done helped create more understanding between network members about their actions.

Reflections on the work

In the initial referral to us, there had been an emphasis on areas of conflict between group-home staff and parents. This made us rather cautious of how best to work with this system. We were influenced by staff views of meetings needing to exclude Sue. In retrospect, though, we may have been over-cautious. We could have undertaken more of the interviewing in mixed network groups together with Sue. However, our individual sessions with Sue provided invaluable insights into her own sense of her dilemma, and we felt in this way able to advocate for her in meetings at which she was not present.

We avoided colluding with different network members about whom or what the problem was. It would have been all too easy to see the problem as "residing" in Sue or her parents, or in either of the different service settings that had failed to provide an interesting enough life for Sue. Instead, through our reflecting conversations we expanded the stories told by focusing on the attitudes and beliefs about the problem held by the different parts of the network. By looking at how these believes affected the communications between the different people involved and what meanings they conveyed, we were able to expand the stories to include new meanings and new solutions to the perceived problems.

Applying theory to practice

Both the above examples are far from blueprints on how to apply systemic practice in group homes. I chose them partly to highlight the many and varied ways in which one might do this work. We may well have achieved the same results following different routes. However, some of the concepts, that I described earlier in this chapter remain central to how I think about the way I work with any particular referral.

In each referral, the "agency life-cycle stage" was considered. This informed our thinking about who needed to be involved in the conversations. In Sue's story, we probably listened too carefully to the initial stories reported by the network! However, the need to consider the context of the referral and what might be expected of the outside agency, and how this fits into the wider systems' expectations and concerns, is important.

In each referral I was mindful of starting with the beliefs and attitudes about the presenting problem. They were obtained in different ways in each of the examples; however, the aim was to uncover the meanings given to the behaviours that had caused the initial referral. By using mainly reflecting processes, enough "news of difference" was introduced to enable the network to move on and to attempt possible new solutions. Most importantly, I tried to avoid providing solutions, attempting instead to remain as a facilitator and co-constructor of new conversations. The key element of this process is some form of network meeting using reflecting-team-style conversations, where the different stories can be heard and made sense of and where client stories are seen as central even if the referred person is not present. As demonstrated, this is not always easy, but without the client as a central person in this process we will remain in a situation where we contribute to creating stories about people which too easily become problem saturated and where the voice of the client remains unheard.+

Who needs to change?

Who you, as the practitioner, think you are when you enter a system is the concept that, to me, provides the main change in emphasis from being a clinical psychologist to being a systemic practitioner. Have you primarily come to solve a problem, or are you there to enable others to solve it? Added to this is one's willingness to be open about what these solutions might be. The system can best judge for itself which solutions are helpful, at any one time. This may not be what you, as a practitioner, anticipated. In this sense, meanings are co-created from the reflections and feedback offered by everyone involved. Nobody's story—not even the practitioner's—is, in theory, prioritized. I see my work as an ongoing series of conversations where the different stories merge and new ones are created. What is seen as helpful may change over time as conversations evolve and as the "meaning-making" process continues.

* * *

Maybe one of the first steps to such changes is in the mind of the practitioner entering these situations. We need to bear in mind our position as *both* the observer *and* the observed, both influencing and being influenced, both part of and outside the systems we are entering. Our willingness to enter without a monopoly on knowledge and information and with openness to possible new interpretations and ways of seeing and acting will, at least partly, determine how differently the issues will be perceived and whether any new meanings, perceptions, and stories emerge. If one is able to make this shift, then working in group homes becomes more of a collaborative exercise where everyone is the expert and their knowledge is valued as important to the process of finding new stories. Having power entails a careful responsibility for how one uses it, which leaves me with my initial question: "Who, indeed, needs to change?"

CHAPTER NINE

The practitioner's position in relation to systemic work in intellectual disability contexts

Helen Pote

As other chapters in this book have shown, systemic models and systemic family therapy offer considerable opportunities to address the emotional and behavioural needs of clients with intellectual disabilities and the systems in which they live. Reports in the literature support this optimism (Fidell, 1996, 2000; Salmon, 1996; Donati, Glynn, Lynggaard, & Pearce, 2000; Gallagher, 2002; Lynggaard & Scior, 2002; Rhodes, 2002, 2003). However, as with any new endeavour, alongside considerable opportunities, clinical dilemmas remain. Some of these dilemmas are general, in that they relate to working with clients whose emotional needs and voice have historically been ignored (Sinason, 1992; Bender, 1993; Wright & Digby, 1996, cited in Caine, Hatton, & Emerson, 1998; Arthur, 1999). Other dilemmas are more specifically related to the application of a systemic model (Rhodes, 2002, 2003). Unfortunately, no therapeutic process or outcome research yet exists in this area to guide practitioners in their decision making and practice.

* * *

This chapter aims to address some of these clinical dilemmas for practitioners, at the levels of theory and practice. Among other things, it discusses how the systemic practitioner addresses the needs of the intellectually disabled client and the wider system. The chapter first considers the context within which practitioners work. It then discusses the clinical dilemmas that commonly arise and how systemic ideas may be useful in addressing these issues.

* * *

The ideas are informed by systemic therapy process research carried out by the author (Pote, 2002, 2004; Pote, Stratton, Cottrell, Shapiro, & Boston, 2003). The arguments presented primarily draw on an interpretative phenomenological analysis (Smith, Jarman, & Osborn, 1999) of interviews with clinical psychologists offering systemic family therapy to clients with intellectual disabilities (Pote, 2002, 2004). The participants in this research were six women and one man, who had been working systemically with people with intellectual disabilities for an average of seven years. The participants had a range of formal systemic training, ranging from multiple systemic workshops to United Kingdom Council for Psychotherapy (UKCP) registration as systemic psychotherapists. The practitioners' accounts referred to throughout the chapter relate to the research interviews conducted by the author. In addition, ideas and examples are drawn from the author's own practice as a clinical psychologist working with children and adults with and without intellectual disabilities. This practice has been influenced by systemic models—particularly Milan and post-Milan (see Campbell, Draper, & Huffington, 1989)—and has involved work with systemic family therapy teams, reflecting teams, and co-therapists, as well as work as a lone therapist. While the ideas from research and practice presented here are based on more traditional, team-based, systemic family therapy, it is acknowledged that systemic practitioners offer a range of interventions to their clients. It is hoped that the ideas in this chapter may also be relevant to dilemmas experienced beyond the boundaries of the therapy room.

* * *

A central tenet of systemic work is to view the difficulties presented, and the client, within a contextual framework (Dallos & Draper, 2000). Contextual models have tried to conceptualize the therapeutic process, by considering the factors that are shaping therapists' practice (Cronen & Pearce, 1985). Such an analysis is crucial for effective systemic work (Clegg, 1993). It enhances opportunities for self-reflexivity. It also offers a systemic framework for considering the practitioner's clinical dilemmas at an intra- and interpersonal level. The following section therefore considers the theoretical and pragmatic contextual influences on practitioners in intellectual disability settings, before turning to clinical dilemmas.

CONTEXTUAL INFLUENCES ON THE SYSTEMIC PRACTITIONER IN INTELLECTUAL DISABILITY SETTINGS

The practitioners who participated in the research pointed to four layers of context that strongly influenced both their views of themselves as therapists and their practice with clients with intellectual disabilities. These contexts were:

- The client with intellectual disabilities.
- The family and wider care system.
- The professional training and service context.
- The social and political environment.

There is obviously overlap and interaction between these contextual layers. The relationships between layers of context are bidirectional, involving both contextual (top-down) and implicative (bottom-up) forces (Cronen & Pearce, 1985). The characteristics of these contextual influences are now described.

The client with intellectual disabilities

The practitioners' accounts emphasized the client-centred focus of their systemic practice. The perspective of the client with intellectual disabilities was central to the practitioners' understanding and practice of systemic therapy and their personal and political motivations for the work more generally. Many practitioners reported feeling both passionate about and dedicated to their work with this client group. They were often motivated by a desire to work with those in most need, within a model that was sensitive to power differentials and cultural factors in society. This emphasis on the needs of the individual with intellectual disabilities is echoed in service models and philosophies, as discussed later.

* * *

The practitioners often emphasized their personal perceptions of people with intellectual disabilities as "people first". They expressed a consistent desire to connect with the client with intellectual disabilities at a very personal and humanistic level. Interestingly, an emphasis on individual identity, above any intellectually disabled identity, has been shown to be associated with positive mental health in people with intellectual disabilities (Finlay & Lyons, 1998). It is also a position consistent with clients' self-perceptions. The majority of people with intellectual disabilities are not likely to label themselves as such (Davies & Jenkins, 1997). In some contexts, they actively position themselves against the label of intellectually disabled, in order to "do being ordinary" (Rapley, Kieman, & Antaki, 1998). Clients therefore are actively co-constructing the reality of themselves as people first. The emphasis on the individual does not imply that practitioners ignore the influence of, and relationships with the immediate carer/family system. However, the importance of the family and wider system is usually viewed as secondary to the needs of the client with an intellectual disability. This is discussed in the next section.

The family and wider care system

In considering the wider family system, the practitioners often expressed concern about the family's unmet economic and emotional needs. Multiple stressors were identified across the family life cycle, including families struggling with loss; difficulties in the transition to adulthood for the intellectually disabled member; the impact of poverty and additional physical health problems; struggles within the parental couple's relationship; and difficulties in the families' relationship with the extended family and professional support services. The rawness of families' emotions in relation to these stressors was often emphasized in practitioners' accounts.

* * *

Literature outlining the characteristics of the family system have emphasized narratives of loss and deficit (for reviews see Byrne & Cunningham, 1985; Vetere, 1993, 1996). There is a consistent theme relating to the family's grief at the "loss of the perfect child" and the re-enactment of this as the child fails to reach a variety of developmental milestones. This literature has influenced systemic practice, with practitioners linking the themes of protection and loss to the family life cycle (Carter & McGoldrick, 1989; Goldberg et al., 1995). Foster (1988) considers the factors that shape such a negative focus in work with families with a member with disability. She suggests that the professional's personal discomfort with the topic of disability might have more influence on this process than families' actual experiences. Such an emphasis on loss and multiple stressors can lead practitioners to align themselves strongly to the client and family, sometimes against the wider system. This positioning often serves a protective function. It may, however, inhibit the development of systemic hypotheses that consider positive discourses regarding coping and resources. The development of literature that uses these more positive discourses may direct therapeutic interventions very differently (Beavers, Hampson, Hulgus, & Beavers, 1986; McConachie, 1993; Dowling & Dolan, 2001).

The professional training and service context

The practitioners' perspectives were also shaped by their professional training and the service contexts within which they practice. The contextual effect of one's professional training consists of both theoretical influences and role expectations. Psychological theories and services relating to people with intellectual disabilities developed at a time when behaviourism was predominant and behaviour modification was the main psychological intervention offered. It was rare that theoretical models or services attended to the emotional needs of clients with intellectual disabilities and their families. The existence of such emotional needs was often denied or marginalized, though the clinical need for such services (in terms of prevalence of mental-health difficulties) was evident (Sinason, 1992; Bender, 1993; Wright & Digby, 1996, cited in Caine, Hatton, & Emerson, 1998; Arthur, 1999; Rhodes, 2002, 2003). Over time, cognitive behavioural (Stenfert Kroese, Dagnan, & Loumidis, 1997) and psychodynamic models and interventions (Sinason, 1992; Waitman & Conboy-Hill, 1992) were offered to this client group. The application of systemic theory and the development of systemic interventions has been slower (Vetere, 1996).

The second aspect of this contextual layer is that of service structures. These include the systemic family therapy team, the community disabilities team, and residential provision. Within this structure, the range of services that are offered to meet the emotional needs of clients still remain patchy. A survey of 80 young people defined as showing challenging behaviour or experiencing a psychiatric disorder found that 64% had received no specialist mental health care as they entered adult services (McCarthy & Boyd, 2002). Statutory and voluntary-sector service structures have developed dichotomies between intellectual disability and mental health services. People with intellectual disabilities and mental health needs, of all ages, often fall through gaps in service provision. This difficulty is particularly acute for children with intellectual disabilities (Gangadharan, Bretherton, & Johnson, 2001; McCarthy & Boyd, 2002). These service structures and the practitioners' relationships with professional colleagues also shape their systemic practice. Difficulties in developing coordinated, collaborative multidisciplinary relationships have been consistently reported for therapeutic services in intellectual disability contexts (Drotar & Sturm, 1996; Risley & Reid, 1996; Caine, Hatton, & Emerson, 1998; Sloper, 1999; Mitchell & Sloper, 2000; Dowling & Dolan, 2001).

The practitioners in the research who worked within existing multidisciplinary services structures reported the need for considerable determination and perseverance in establishing systemic services for clients with intellectual disabilities. However, their experience of working with the systemic therapy team was overwhelmingly positive. Practitioners often viewed the team as a resource for both personal and professional development.

The social and political environment

The final contextual influence on the practitioners who participated in the research was the wider societal and political environment. This consisted of structural components such as service capacity and priorities, as well as ideological components such as service philosophies and societal perceptions of people with intellectual disabilities.

* * *

There have been many developments over the past three decades in models of both residential and day-care services for people with intellectual disabilities (Department of Health & Social Security, 1971; Mittler & Sinason, 1996, cited in Caine, Hatton, & Emerson, 1998). These changes have been influenced by a range of service philosophies, such as normalization (Wolfensberger, 1972; O'Brien, 1987) and community care (Department of Health, 1992). Many of these philosophies have assumed an individualized, and sometimes medicalized, view of the needs of people with intellectual disabilities. They have rarely explicitly considered relational or systemic models (McIntosh, 2002).

Resource and policy limitations had a strong contextual impact on systemic work with people with intellectual disabilities. These shaped the family's and practitioners' experience of the wider professional system and also their interactions with this system in their therapeutic work. For example, practitioners were often angered by the wider professional-system limitations, such as the lack of respite-care provision. This limited their ability to facilitate change through therapy itself.

* * *

Societal perceptions of people with intellectual disabilities also inform this context. These perceptions have largely been negative. For example, when a lay population was asked to assess the connotations they associated with recent and historical labels for intellectual disabilities, they rated all labels, apart from "exceptional", as having negative connotations. Those members of the public who knew someone with an intellectual disability rated the terms more negatively than those who had no personal experience of someone with such difficulties (Hastings, Sonuga-Barke, & Remington, 1996).

* * *

In summary, the four contextual influences discussed above provide a systemic framework within which we can understand the dilemmas faced by practitioners working systemically with this client group. In the next section, I outline some of these dilemmas in detail and discuss how systemic ideas may be helpful in addressing them. Examples from practice are used to illustrate these ideas.

CLINICAL DILEMMAS AND SYSTEMIC RESPONSES

Practitioners' position in relation to the client, family, and wider system: the struggle to stay curious

A key dilemma for the practitioners in the research was how to position themselves in relation to the client, family, and wider system. The primary influence of the client with intellectual disabilities, and practitioners' concerns about how the wider system was meeting the client's needs, often led practitioners to align themselves with the client and/or family and remain distant or opposed to the wider system.

The practitioners' position was perhaps consolidated by their personal motivations for working with those in most need, coupled with the intra- and interpersonal conflicts posed by being both "part of" and critical or distant from the wider professional system.

Such positions can be justified as being consistent with service philosophies that give political weight to the primacy of the intellectually disabled client. This is demonstrated in partnership models of intellectual disabilitiy services (*Valuing People*: Department of Health, 2001) and advocacy models such as that proposed by People First (People First, 1995). Recent systemic models have also tried to empower people whose views may have been subjugated by the systems within which they function (White & Epston, 1990) and so may also be used to justify the practitioner's close alignment with the client.

This alignment to the client or family often serves a protective function. A triangular pattern of protection between practitioners, parents, and the person with intellectual disabilities is common, with each person trying to protect the others from emotional or physical distress (Goldberg et al., 1995; Pote, King, & Clegg, 2004). For example, parents may try to protect their adult son or daughter with intellectual disabilities from risk factors inherent in independent living. The person with intellectual disabilities may strive to protect his or her parents from feelings of responsibility and try to care for their physical needs as they grow older. The practitioners also participates in this protective triangle. They often serve as the protector of the human rights of the individual with intellectual disabilities—for example, as a person entitled to make choices and take risks.

This triangle of protection sometimes brings tensions and feelings of anger in the protectors, as they can feel that their protective strategies are becoming ineffective. This can easily turn into a blaming stance towards the person being protected or others in the system. This triangle of protection, and the associated feelings of anger and blame, could be usefully connected to the general relationship struggles and patterns of criticism that commonly develop between families, therapists, and the wider system. I shall return to ideas for facilitating this therapeutic process shortly.

Given the existence of these tensions, it is clear that the practitioners' close alignment with the client with intellectual disabilities may bring dilemmas for them when they are trying to work systemically. How can they be systemic, and maintain a curious and non-blaming attitude towards all system members, while also emphasizing the needs of those in most need or at most risk of being silenced? This dilemma is perhaps most acute when the voice of the client with intellectual disabilities is clearly being ignored.

* * *

The general systemic literature has explored the issue of alignment using the concepts of neutrality (Selvini Palazzoli, Boscolo, Cecchin, & Prata, 1980) and later curiosity (Cecchin, 1987). These ideas emphasize the even-handed position that practitioners should take in relation to all members of the system, while also acknowledging the need to address power differences. Various strategies have been suggested for practitioners to enable them to maintain their curious and even-handed stance.

Central to these strategies is the idea of the practitioners' reflexivity—that is, their capacity to monitor and reflect upon their own actions and emotions. Self-reflexivity focuses especially on the effect of the therapy process upon the practitioner and the way in which this is a resource for change in his or her work with the family (Flaskas & Perlesz, 1996). In order to use self-reflexivity, it is necessary for practitioners to be alert and irreverent to their own constructions, functioning, and prejudices, so that they can use themselves effectively with the family (Cecchin, Lane, & Ray, 1992).

Reflexivity also connects to practitioners' personal and political motivations for the work. These motivations appear particularly passionate in intellectual disability contexts and relate to a desire to empower those in most need. Recently, narrative therapists have discussed the importance of therapists bringing their personal motivations and development into the therapeutic conversations with clients (White, 1995, 1997, 2000). This facilitates a two-way account of therapy as affecting both client and therapist. It also empowers clients and therapists by emphasizing the resources each are bringing to the therapy process (White, 1997).

This reflective discussion may be particularly helpful for practitioners working within intellectual disability contexts where the work may be devalued due to societal negative influences and can provoke feelings of disablement in the practitioner and client (Goldberg et al., 1995). As the feelings of disablement may hinder the occurrence of this reflexive process, it may therefore be helpful for the practitioner and family to utilize reflecting-team methods (Andersen, 1991) to develop reflexivity.

* * *

The "problem-determined system" is a further systemic idea that may be helpful in addressing this alignment dilemma. Given the earlier discussion regarding triangles of protection, it will obviously be important for practitioners to develop a clear understanding of the relationship each system member has to each of the others, to the presenting difficulties, and to the practitioner themselves. Mapping the "problem-determined system" is clearly relevant to practitioners trying to achieve this task (Anderson & Goolishian, 1986). The problem-determined system describes the people that connect to the presenting problem and how they affect it and are organized by it. Resolution of the difficulties will therefore result in dissolution of the problem-determined system.

* * *

In intellectual disability contexts, the mapping of the problem-determined system and the relationships that exist within it could be achieved by taking a systemic approach to network meetings, involving client, family, carers, practitioner, and referrer at the beginning of the systemic work. Bloomfield, Nielsen, and Kaplan (1984) suggest how to neutrally address conflicts between the family and wider care system in intellectual disability contexts. Their ideas include the development of a "decisional subsystem" and the sharing of systemic ideas and formulations with the system. This might mitigate against some of the alignment dilemmas I have discussed.

* * *

Systemic models of consultation (see Selma Rikberg Smyly, chapter 8) may also prove helpful in enabling practitioners to remain neutral and to relate with increased curiosity in their relationships with the wider system. General systemic models of consultation have suggested how practitioners can understand and work effectively with the wider system by using the core concept of the organizational life cycle (Campbell, Draper, & Huffington, 1991; Campbell, 1995, 2000). They propose that organizational change and new ideas will be interpreted according to the system's and individual member's existing sets of beliefs and assumptions. They reflect on the conflicts that may exist between ideas that are held by the system and those held by its individual members. Successful change in the wider system is therefore facilitated by developing the connections between individuals' belief sets (Campbell, 1995). As contacts with other professionals in intellectual disability contexts are often brief, frequent, and informal, such consultation models will need to be adapted to establish an effective systemic liaison or brief consultation (Mason, 1991; Street & Downey, 1996).

* * *

In the following example from my own practice, I illustrate how practitioners may maintain a curious and systemic stance towards their relationships to the problem, the client, the family, and wider system. This process is aided by taking a reflexive approach to supervision and mapping the problem-determined system.

John

John is 39 years old, with moderate intellectual disabilities and epilepsy. He has lived with his younger brother, Trevor, since his parents died eight years ago. The relationship between the brothers has not been easy, and Trevor now has serious health problems. Trevor appears to treat his brother as a child, and at home John has little opportunity to make choices and decisions. Recently Trevor has suggested that John move to live with his aunt, Margaret. John seems happy with this, but he is being given little opportunity to participate in the decision-making process by his family. John's social worker feels that John may be better placed in a supported-living project so he has opportunities to develop his independence. The social worker refers John to the clinical psychologist for work to facilitate him in making choices about his residential provision. She feels that John needs a stronger voice and a chance to express choice in his family. The practitioner's initial reaction is that, as an adult, John has a right to make choices about his living situation, and facilitating the expression and fulfilment of these choices is primary.

Clinical dilemma

How can practitioners address their initial assumptions about the referral and their close alignment with the position of the client and social worker? There is a risk that practitioners may lose the capacity to conceptualize the referral systemically, thus aligning themselves with the client/professionals against the family system.

Systemic responses

Self-reflexivity. Reflecting on the origins of clinical assumptions in order to maintain curiosity was important for the practitioner in this situation. The question of how to approach the referral was taken to a supervision session. This was organized systemically, with one member of the team interviewing the lead practitioner about his or her ideas and assumptions in relation to this referral. The other members of the supervision group had a reflecting conversation about these in front of the lead practitioner. Among other ideas, they expressed a concern about facilitating John to express his views outside the family context, without a discussion of how decisions were negotiated in the culture of this family. They felt that this may not be empowering for John or his family, in developing joint decision making.

Defining the problem-determined system. The task for the practitioner in responding systemically to this referral was to try to find ways to include and appreciate the perspectives of all system members that are connected to and affected by the residential decision (John, Trevor, Margaret, and the social worker). In effect, this was the decisional subsystem. A network meeting was proposed by the practitioner, with all family members and the referrer attending. The meeting was used to clarify consent for the referral from John and to explore what each person hoped to achieve from the work. This was conducted using circular questions to allow everyone the opportunity to express their views and comment on the views expressed by others. Some family and individual sessions were offered following this to explore themes of decision making and to enable John to express his views.

Inclusion of the client with intellectual disabilities

The majority of the systemic practitioners in my research emphasized their commitment to a positive and collaborative therapy process. They often discussed the need to facilitate inclusion of all system members, and they made efforts to concretize the process of therapy to meet the needs of the client with intellectual disabilities. The theme of inclusion is echoed in the socio-political context (*Valuing People*: Department of Health, 2001). Ideas of inclusion also connect to a focus in the wider systemic literature about effectively including the less articulate members of the family in the therapeutic process (White & Epston, 1990;

Wilson, 1998a). The aim of inclusion itself seems consistent with systemic practice and is relatively unproblematic. Dilemmas arise mainly when practitioners are concerned that, although their clients with intellectual disabilities are included in the process of family therapy, their full potential for participation is not achieved. Systemic family therapy, like most psychological interventions, is often reliant on verbal participation, some degree of abstract thinking, and the mapping of themes or relationships across time. It is important for systemic models to conceptualize inclusion as extending beyond the process of therapy sessions. Systemic practitioners may need to revise their theories, models of practice, and definitions of participation to shift the focus away from verbal interactions and abstract relational concepts.

An example of the need for such revision can be seen in the model of narrative therapy developed by White and Epston (1990), which is based on an analysis of power and its effects on individuals' lives. The process of therapy they outline uses the metaphor of narrative, and the ability to develop new narratives through the therapeutic conversation, as central to change in interactions and behaviour. Within their theoretical model and therapy process, language is privileged above other forms of shared action. This may considerably exclude those without sophisticated language skills from participating fully in shaping constructions. People with intellectual disabilities are not often skilled discourse users, and thus such a focus on language-based change may contribute to further disempowering them and decreasing their ability to "warrant voice" within society (Burr, 1995). Such models need to be carefully adapted to emphasize other forms of shared action and meaning making (e.g., behaviour and nonverbal communication) if we are to extend narrative models to incorporate the needs of people with intellectual disabilities. Systemic practitioners in intellectual disability settings have made significant recent progress in adapting the process of narrative therapy to meet the needs of their clients (see Katrina Scior & Henrik Lynggaard, chapter 6). However, further critical analysis of the underlying theoretical model is warranted to develop its applicability to those whose primary means of communicating are not through language (Pote, 2001).

In addition, systemic practitioners unused to working with the needs of people with intellectual disabilities need to be challenged about their marginalization of this client group. Often this marginalization is based on the hypothesis that intellectually disabled clients require specific therapeutic skills to facilitate inclusion, skills that are above and beyond the skills of mainstream systemic practitioners (Rhodes, 2002). This hypothesis may explain the service dichotomies discussed earlier. It would be helpful to use other hypotheses that emphasize the commonalities in working systemically across client groups and use systemic ideas to facilitate integrated service planning (see Sabrina Halliday and Lorna Robbins, chapter 3).

Relationship to help

One particular tension for the practitioners in my research was how they viewed the model of change and the client's relationship to help in intellectual disability contexts. The relationship to therapeutic and other services was often ongoing, and practitioners noted the struggle for themselves and families in ending therapy. This may relate to the persistence of difficulties throughout the life cycle, inherent in, and associated with, the intellectual disabilities. The struggle to end therapy may also relate to particular family life-cycle issues common for this client group, such as difficulties in establishing independence for both parents and children (Turnbull, Summers, & Brotherson, 1986). To address these dilemmas, we need to question the primary purpose of therapy as being towards promoting change. It may be necessary to integrate support across the life cycle into one's model of change. This will prevent an ongoing relationship to therapeutic services being pathologized, and it could redefine the way the beginnings and endings of therapy are conceptualized. Fredman and Dalal (1998) have considered ending issues in systemic therapy, and they suggest ways to end therapy that empower families to draw upon their own resources in the future. Reder and Fredman (1996) have also considered families' relationship to help and explored how practitioners' and families' beliefs about the treatment process interact from the first therapeutic contact and should be explored in detail. Supervision could help practitioners to map their own and the families' models of change. Defining successful outcomes at the start of therapy would promote self-reflexivity and may be helpful in empowering practitioners and families in successful conclusion to their therapeutic relationship. Techniques from solution-focused models, such as "the miracle question", may be helpful in facilitating these conversations (de Shazer, 1985).

* * *

In the following example from my own practice, I want to illustrate how practitioners can utilize systemic ideas to examine and understand their relationships with clients and families and the wider system. This understanding may enrich their work with families by addressing obstacles that could affect the collaborative therapeutic relationships. It may also offer new perspectives to the family in order that they might develop their own reflective processes.

Rabeya and Fayek

Rabeya (10 years) and her brother Fayek (12 years) live at home with their mother, Mrs Ali. Both children have mild intellectual disabilities. They are active and eager to interact with their peers. The children attend a local special-needs school and are able to undertake many tasks independently—for example, both can follow directions in a classroom setting and can dress themselves at home. Mrs Ali finds it difficult to manage their active behaviour at home. Their father has contact with the family, but this is rather irregular due to work commitments that take him abroad for long periods. The children and their mother have been attending systemic family therapy sessions with the community team for over a year. During this time they have begun to think about the development of independence for the children and Mrs Ali, and Mrs Ali's confidence in her parenting has increased considerably. The practitioner had planned a final appointment with the family. However, Mrs Ali cancelled the appointment, as the children's father was back in the UK. Some weeks later she contacted the clinic asking for urgent help in managing the children's behaviour as their father had now returned to working abroad.

Clinical dilemma

How can the practitioner respond systemically to the family's request for further help in a manner that both sensitively addresses their current concerns and emphasizes the progress and resources they have developed over the therapeutic relationship?

Systemic responses

Understanding their relationship to help. In addressing the dilemma, it was useful for the practitioner to consider in supervision what relationship the family may have to help. This assisted the practitioner in questioning how this was affected by the family's cultural contexts, particularly what the culturally acceptable ways were to offer and receive help. Within this, the practitioner also came to understand the roles both they and the father were taking in relation to the family developing both independence and their own resources. Did Mrs Ali, for instance, have a narrative about the family needing life-long support from a partner or agency? These ideas helped the practitioner and the team to offer another therapy session. They reviewed the current difficulties but then focused on the theme of endings and past/future relationships to helpers, which may build on existing strengths and resources rather than replace them.

Practitioners' relationship to an expert position

For all the practitioners I interviewed, there was a clear dilemma about giving advice and being perceived or positioned by families and other professionals as an expert. The dilemma of taking the expert position and imparting specific and directive communications to the family is one that the field of systemic therapy has struggled with for some time (Maturana, 1988; Silver, 1991). The giving of advice is regarded by some systemic practitioners as poor practice. This is despite the fact that it has been suggested that advice correlates with clients' positive view of their therapist and with a successful therapeutic outcome for systemic family therapy (Bennun, 1989).

In intellectual disability contexts, this dilemma is often more frequent and acute. This may be attributed to a number of factors. Practitioners have been traditionally positioned in an expert position by behavioural and diagnostic models that paid scant attention to the positions or views of the client (Anderson & Goolishian, 1992; Arthur, 1999). In addition, this work was often conducted indirectly, through carers, with practitioners taking an advisory role and issues of consent to treatment largely ignored. Interactions with the wider system also sometimes require the practitioner to offer an expert opinion—for example, participation in the statementing process to enable children with intellectual disabilities to access appropriate educational resources. These role expectations and the fact that practitioners are working with clients who have more limited ability and opportunity to make choices (Lancioni, O'Reilly, & Emerson, 1996) intensify practitioners' concerns about taking an expert position. The socio-political context of discrimination, equality, and normalization for people with intellectual disabilities increases the necessity of an equal and collaborative relationship with clients.

* * *

In offering systemic family therapy, the dilemma for the practitioners I interviewed seemed to be focused on the ethical concerns raised by what were seen as first-order normative and directive systemic models, such as structural therapy (Minuchin, 1974; Minuchin & Fishman, 1981). Many practitioners expressed a strong desire to move away from structural models of therapy in an attempt to develop a more collaborative, non-expert relationship with clients. However, they also recognized the strengths of some of the structural techniques, such as enactment, in engaging their client group in concrete demonstrations of the relational difficulties they experience.

* * *

Models for developing eclectic systemic practice may help practitioners in intellectual disability contexts formulate and work collaboratively using more recent systemic ideas, while drawing on more traditional systemic techniques. Burnham (1992) proposed a model to facilitate integration both across systemic models and with other psychological models. This "approach–method–technique" model discusses three levels guiding therapists' practice:

1. *approach*—the assumptions, values, theoretical ideas, and ethical stance held by the therapist;
2. *method*—the working practices and organizational patterns shaping practice;
3. *techniques*—the individual activities and tools used by the lead practitioner and the team.

Within this framework, particular ideas can be considered within or across the levels of a systemic approach, method, or technique. A practitioner may therefore formulate a family's difficulties using a systemic approach but utilize a behavioural technique. Flaskas (2000) has suggested such eclecticism will enhance systemic thought and practice by emphasizing continuities between systemic ideas and by being more closely representative of the complex demands of therapeutic practice.

* * *

Introducing reflecting-team models into practice may also be helpful in responding to dilemmas about taking an expert position. Reflecting teams arise from a social constructionist framework, where truths are questioned and ideas and concepts are viewed as discourses that are in competition for prevalence and importance (dominance) in society's construction of reality (Foucault, 1980; Dallos & Draper, 2000). Within such a framework, an expert view or position would be understood as one that had gained prominence or power but was not necessarily the true or correct position. The reflecting-team process aims to introduce the new and multiple ideas into the therapeutic conversation in a reflexive manner (Andersen, 1991). There are many different forms that reflexive discussion may take, and these are adapted to suit the wishes and needs of the family in therapy. Consistently, the family are asked both to reflect on the ways in which the ideas offered by the reflecting team connect to their own thinking and to discuss how it would be helpful to take these ideas forward into the conversation with the practitioner.

In the following example from my practice, I illustrate how systemic ideas and working practices facilitate a collaborative working relationship with clients that helpfully addresses issues of power and expertise. This serves to empower clients with intellectual disabilities and their families.

Olga

Olga is an 18-year-old woman with moderate intellectual disabilities and challenging behaviour, which includes physical aggression towards her peers. She has been excluded from two of her three school placements. The current placement is working well, but Olga's family and current teachers are concerned about organizing an appropriate day-placement for when she leaves school next year. The family have been coming to family therapy sessions for some time to think about how best to manage the challenging behaviours as a family and for Olga to develop her independence. The sessions have been characterized by the parents asking the practitioner for advice on the best way to manage these concerns. They come to a session one day with information from the local social-services department regarding day centres, and they ask the practitioner if she could make an assessment of which provision would best meet Olga's needs.

Clinical dilemmas

How can the practitioner share her ideas and opinions while working collaboratively with Olga and her family and enhancing their confidence in their own expertise and ability to make choices?

Systemic responses

The practitioner was very concerned not to position herself as an expert when a variety of choices may be appropriate for the family. She also held the view that Olga and her family would be the best assessor of which day provision was appropriate, feeling that the family could most effectively evaluate which day-care facilities were most consistent with their beliefs, values, and desires. However, the practitioner was also aware that she held a lot of knowledge about local day-care facilities which may be helpful to the family. Therefore, after interviewing the family about the day-service options available to them and their current thinking and decision making, the practitioner suggested that the therapy team offer ideas using a reflecting-team format.

A theme that was discussed by the team was the family's natural concern to "get things right" and the parent's struggle to trust their own and Olga's views within this decision-making process. They highlighted the idea that there might not be one right choice and discussed how the choice would be different for different people and would change over time. They talked about the decision-making style in the family and how this process had developed as Olga grew older and how it would change into her adult years. The team ended by acknowledging their dilemma of whether offering their opinions on day care would help or hinder the family in the development of the family's own decision-making capacity.

Following this, the practitioner asked the family which ideas had resonated with them and which they would like to take forward in their conversation with the practitioner. The parents said they were concerned about whether Olga would be happy with the choices they were being asked to make and felt it would be helpful to think about ways to include Olga more in the decision making, perhaps using the sessions to do this. Olga looked pleased with the conversation but did not add any comment.

CONCLUSIONS

Systemic interventions and systemic family therapy offer a great deal of promise in meeting the needs of clients with intellectual disabilities and their systems. As with any exciting development, it is important for practitioners to pause and carefully consider the dilemmas they face when applying a new model. This chapter has aimed to outline the dilemmas associated with a systemic model and offer ideas that may be useful in furthering systemic practice with this client group.

* * *

It is clear that more specific research regarding the process and efficacy of systemic family therapy with clients with intellectual disabilities is needed in order to satisfy the demands of clinical governance and the evidenced-based culture of clinical psychology services (Roth & Fonagy, 1996) as well as to develop an ethical service for our clients. Given the paucity of the systemic research base in intellectual disability contexts, this will not be an easy process. This is further complicated by issues of both capacity and consent that have impeded traditional randomized controlled trials in intellectual disability contexts (Oliver et al., 2002). Nevertheless such evaluations are urgently needed if family therapy is to continue to be offered alongside more long-standing interventions.

* * *

It would be useful to conduct further research to explore any solutions that practitioners have generated in response to the intra- and interpersonal conflicts and dilemmas posed by systemic work in intellectual disability contexts. In addition, understanding the experience of the systemic family therapy process from client and family perspectives (such as Arkless, 2005) will help the development of an interactional research base regarding the process of systemic family therapy with people with intellectual disabilities. Services need to consider a systemic model in developing services and addressing dilemmas. At the core will be a reflexive approach to practice that is responsive to client feedback and is inclusive at the levels of theory and practice in considering the needs of all system members.

Key learning points

- A systemic approach to working with clients with intellectual disabilities offers considerable promise but also poses certain dilemmas for practitioners.
- When working systemically with clients with intellectual disabilities, it is important to understand the work within a systemic contextual framework.
- Practitioners' accounts pointed to four layers of context that influenced their views of themselves as practitioners and their practice with clients with intellectual disabilities:
    —the client with intellectual disabilities
    —the family and wider care system
    —the professional training and service context
    —the social and political environment.
- These contextual influences interact in a bidirectional manner, exerting both contextual (top-down) and implicative (bottom-up) forces that shape the therapeutic work with clients.
- Key dilemmas for systemic practitioners in these contexts included:
    —the practitioners' position in relation to the client with intellectual disabilities, the family, and the wider system.
    —the inclusion of people with intellectual disabilities
    —the systems relationship to help
    —the practitioners' relationship to an expert position.
- Systemic ideas such as self-reflexivity, contextualizing practice, identifying problem-determined systems, and understanding the clients' relationship to help may be useful to practitioners in addressing these dilemmas.

CHAPTER TEN

So how do I . . . ?

Henrik Lynggaard and Sandra Baum

Overview

The contributors to this book have shown many different ways in which systemic approaches can be used and adapted when working with people affected by intellectual disabilities. We know from our own experiences that while a good grounding in the theories that inform any therapeutic approach is invaluable, it is often practical questions of the type *"How do I . . . ?"* and *"How can I . . . ?"* that occupy the practitioner as she or he explores the usefulness or relevance of a different approach. Many of the contributors have shared their experiences of beginning to incorporate systemic approaches into their practice, and we thought it would be useful to summarize some of the contributors' practical suggestions in one place, adding further ideas where appropriate. We have done this under the heading of a series of questions that some readers might have.

How can I get started?

Individual practitioner's circumstances and work settings will vary widely and present different opportunities and constraints. Though it is unlikely that a given service model will translate neatly to a different context, a number of contributors to this book describe the journey they embarked on in establishing a systemic service. Some of their ideas may be of relevance to others. For example, Sandra Baum and Sarah Walden (chapter four) provide a six-point guide to establishing a systemic service in a community team for people with intellectual disabilities. Among other things they suggest that practitioners identify colleagues with a similar interest, access supervision, adopt a step-wise approach, and audit their work as they go along. In Baum and Walden's own words:

- Make contact with colleagues within your context who are interested in working systemically.
- "Audit" your systemic knowledge, experience, and interest—you may be pleasantly surprised by what you find!
- Access systemic supervision—there may be someone within your wider service setting, or professional groups, who is willing to supervise you or at least have initial conversations with you about your ideas.
- Start small—identify one or two examples of work where a systemic approach may be appropriate, to allow you to develop your confidence.
- Keep managers informed about what you are doing—they may be able to let you know if there are any monies available for supervision costs, training, and so forth.
- Evaluate your work—it shows managers that working systemically is worthwhile.

Sabrina Halliday and Lorna Robbins (chapter three) demonstrate how teaming up across different specialities can create an innovative lifespan service. They also share their experiences of establishing a systemic service through a number of practical suggestions:

- If you are a small service, working across the lifespan may be the most feasible and cost-effective way of delivering family therapy.
- Consider where your team would fit in with local need and other service provision and ensure that you are part of the system and are supported by it.
- Find interested people in key service areas who use systemic approaches for support, discussion, and development.
- Obtain and maintain management agreement and support for working in this way—for example, lifespan family therapy teams meet *Valuing People* (Department of Health, 2001) and *National Service Framework* (Department of Health, 1999) targets for working with carers as well as service users.
- Apply the model to yourself in working practices (e.g., training, supervision, research).
- Audit, evaluate and disseminate work to others (and be prepared to write about it).
- Involve students and trainees: as well as helping with evaluation, they have fresh perspectives to offer families and teams.
- Involve service users in the development of the service.
- Keep inspired (e.g., networking, training days, away-days).

* * *

Fortunately—and as Glenda Fredman demonstrates in her own practice (chapter one)—one does not need to establish a family or systemic service with one-way mirror, cameras, and teams in order to draw on systemic approaches. As shown in the next section, there are many other ways of using and incorporating the ideas in one's practice.

How do I apply systemic ideas in my work setting?

Bill was the only psychologist working in a multidisciplinary community team for people with intellectual disabilities. Medical models, or models that viewed the individual client as the main site of intervention, tended to hold dominance. Bill was keen to use some of the ideas and practices that had excited him while undertaking a systemic training course, but for a while he could not identify any colleagues with a shared interest in the social constructionist ideas that had stirred his own enthusiasm. Bill decided that he would begin his systemic practice by asking questions. When it felt appropriate he would ask these questions in referral meetings, in discussions about clients, and in his conversation on the phone with referrers. He grew fond of a range of questions along the lines of: "Whose idea was it to refer Michael to our service?" "What, I wonder, might they have had in mind for Michael?" "Who else is significant in Michael's life?" "What ideas or views might Michael have about all this?" "What do you think Michael would say if he had been listening to our conversation?" and so forth. In asking such questions, it was Bill's intention to provide a relational focus, to invite multiple perspectives, and to try to invite discussion about the views of the person with intellectual disabilities.

As has been suggested, drawing on systemic approaches in one's practice does not necessarily require a particular physical setting, technical apparatus, a team, or all the key people in the system to be present. The approach and its associated methods and techniques can be used in shaping many aspects of work. For example, it can be used to inform conversations and interactions with individuals, with families, with staff teams and networks and in supervision and training. At the risk of oversimplification, it could be argued that one of the key skills of the systemic practitioner consists in asking questions that keep a relational focus and that invite many voices to join and be heard. Among these, "Who" questions can be particularly useful—"Who is concerned?" "Who is involved?" "Who has a view?" "Who is affected?"—and so on. As Fredman (personal communication 2000) has said, metaphorically such "Who" questions "people" the space or room. These relational practices are also what make it entirely possible to use a systemic approach with individuals. Examples of working with individuals but drawing in the wider system either through the questions that are asked or through broadening the network of people in conversation with each other, are given by Katrina Scior and Henrik Lynggaard (chapter six). Selma Rikberg Smyly (chapter eight) describes the application of systemic approaches when working with staff teams in group homes. In another context Lynggaard, Donati, Pearce, and Sklavounos (2002) describe how a systemic approach may influence the discussion of referrals in a multidisciplinary setting. Dixon and Matthews (1992), as well as Helen Pote (chapter nine), show how systemic ideas may be used in peer supervision and to enable reflective practice when discussing complex situations.

How do I decide when to use a systemic approach?

For us a systemic *approach* provides a framework for all of our practice, even when we undertake activities that do not require specific systemic *methods* or *techniques*. For instance, as psychologists we are often asked to undertake psychometric testing, our speech therapist colleagues might be asked to undertake a swallowing assessment, or a medical colleague might be asked to prescribe medication. None of these tasks immediately suggests systemic methods and techniques, but each could be approached systemically by an appreciation of the context in which the task is taking place, the relationships that have led to the requests, and the nature of the relationships between the particular service, the professional, and the client.

When using a systemic approach, we have found that systemic methods and techniques have a positive contribution to make to the following situations:

- When people ask to be seen together.
- When the issue referred is identified as relational (e.g., "John and his mother are having repeated arguments").
- When there is a primary problem that is not immediately seen as relational (e.g., autism), but relationships are significantly affected by or affecting the problem.
- Where families or others in the network offer a potential resource to the resolution of the problem.

How do I decide when to see people together?

As Fredman (chapter one) has pointed out, using a systemic approach does not automatically imply seeing people together, and there are many examples in this book of working systemically with individuals.

Therefore, questions may arise for practitioners about who to include in the work and whether or not to see people together or separately. When deciding who the system in focus is, we have found helpful guidance in the questions suggested by Lang and McAdam (1995): "Who is concerned?" "Who is involved?" "Who is significant?" We have found these questions particularly useful in making decisions about whom to invite to sessions.

* * *

When making decisions about whom to include in the work we also consider:

- Does the family/significant network understand or agree with the invitation to be seen together?
- Is there a risk that an invitation to be seen together might be perceived by the family/network as criticizing or blaming?
- If you are regarded as a family therapy service, are there any other professionals working with the family? If so, will it be confusing for the family to be invited to meet with you? Are the other familiar professionals already doing the work, or could they do the work with your support?

We have found the following, perhaps more obvious points particularly useful when deciding not to invite people to be seen in the same room together:

- When people decline to be seen together.
- When the person clearly requests being seen alone.
- Where there is a high level of risk associated with bringing people together.
- When a different kind of help is needed (e.g., the family may not want a therapist and three reflecting-team members to arrive in response to a request for help in completing a housing-application form!).

It is perhaps worth re-emphasizing that a systemic approach also lends itself to working with different combinations of a given system at different times. Several contributors to this book have referred to situations where a decision was made to, for example, meet with the person with intellectual disabilities on his or her own for a few sessions. They found that these sessions could allow extra time for the person to express his or her ideas or for the practitioners and the person to tune into and attune their respective ways of communicating.

How do I include people with intellectual disabilities?

All of the authors in this book express what Helen Pote in chapter nine terms, "a consistent desire to connect with the client with intellectual disabilities". But as she goes on to argue the question arises of how the practitioner can "maintain a curious and non-blaming attitude towards all system members, while also emphasizing the needs of those in most need or at most risk of being silenced ... [especially] when the voice of the client with intellectual disabilities is clearly being ignored." Contributors have offered a range of ideas and practical suggestions for including and giving voice to people. There are, of course, no hard and fast rules that will guide the practitioner in all situations, and we frequently remind ourselves that people who are subsumed under the description of "intellectual disabilities" comprise a heterogeneous group with very varied abilities and needs. One cannot, therefore, be prescriptive and can only offer some suggestions to act as guidance. Importantly, ideas and practices that facilitate participation can also be drawn from the systemic literature on working with other groups where there are barriers to full inclusion such as working with children (Wilson, 1998a), with people with sensory impairments, or with people with memory problems (Sabat, 2001). Many skills and knowledges, gained in working with different client groups, may also as Halliday and Robbins's colleagues discovered, transfer to working with people affected with intellectual disabilities. What follows is a list of suggestions that have emerged through practices described both in this book and elsewhere. We are aware that we sometimes touch briefly on some big issues, and that some of our suggestions, in turn, invite further questions and debate.

Enabling participation. One of the key responsibilities of the systemic practitioner is to create space for participation for the person with intellectual disabilities. It may require minimal adaptations of language and style to join in conversations with people affected by milder degrees of intellectual disabilities. However, the practitioner may be severely challenged when communication in its broadest forms is limited or inconsistent and when intent is ambiguous. In those circumstances, meanings may emerge only slowly and over time and in a weaving backwards and forwards between the person and those who know him or her well. While such a view of meanings as socially constructed between individuals is coherent with some of the theories that inform systemic approaches, the practitioner needs to be mindful of how differences in power can operate to fix or freeze meaning in ways that could further disadvantage people. Participation and inclusion are enabled when the practitioner and those who join him or her are able to remain curious and patient, are willing to struggle with uncertainty, and can voice questions that invite the possibility of people being "heard".

People with severe and profound intellectual disabilities. Writing in a different context, Iveson (1990) suggests a way of inviting and imagining the voice of a person with no speaking voice and a very severe degree of disabilities. The process Iveson proposes involves asking a series of questions that invite people to adopt, or to speak from, a different position—for example: *"If Saleha could speak and if I were to ask her to choose someone to speak for her at this meeting, who do you think she would choose?"* A discussion may follow among participants about which choice the person would make, which in itself may be helpful. Iveson suggests further questions along the following lines, where the "me" refers to Iveson and Muni refers to Saleha's sister:

"*Me*: So, Muni, will you agree to be Saleha's "voice" for this meeting?

Muni: Yes.

Me: Well, what I'd like you to do is when I want to ask Saleha a question, I want you to answer as if you were Saleha. Will you be able to do that?

Muni: But I might not be able to get it right.

Me: No, I'm sure you won't get it right all the time because you're a different person, but I'd still like you to do it. Will you?

Muni: Yes.

Me: It will mean that sometimes you'll have to speak twice, once for Saleha and once for yourself. [*Everyone laughs.*] [Iveson, 1990, pp. 82–83]

The therapeutic intent in such an approach is to invite people to stand in and relate from a different position, a position that may otherwise become marginalized. Centring a position in this way may open up new understanding and opportunities for action. Out of this speaking, listening, and reflecting, a criss-crossing of perspectives may arise within which new ideas can emerge.

Lending the words. Booth and Booth (1996) describe a process of occasionally offering or lending people the words with which to participate in their research. They developed a series of successive approximations trying out different words that may fit for people. An example of this from our own practice shows one way in which this may be used. Frank was a man in his mid-30s with a mild to moderate degree of intellectual disabilities and was seen for individual work by the first author [HL]. As the example indicates, Frank sometimes struggled to find the words to express and to communicate his experiences. In the episode referred to below, he had been describing how he would frequently punch his fist against the wall, so that it became bruised and swollen:

Frank: "I don't know what it is. I don't know what it is. Something up there, something up there [*pointing to his head*] makes me do it. I don't know what it is . . ."

HL: "Something up there, in your head, makes you do it?"

Frank: "Yes, I don't know what it is. Something in here [*pointing*] makes me do it?"

HL: "Does the 'something in there' have another name or names?"

Frank: "I don't know what it is. But something makes me do it?"

HL: "Would you be interested in knowing more about what it is? . . . In finding out if it is connected to other things?"

Frank: "Yes, but I don't know what it is. Something makes me do it. Something up there [*again points to his head*]."

HL: "When you punch your fist against the wall, you hurt yourself.

And you have told me that you don't like hurting yourself. That you would like to stop it? Is that right?"

Frank: "Yes. Yes, but I don't know what makes me do it."

HL: "So at the moment, it is not clear what makes you do it. Do you think that the 'something' is connected to things that have happened to you?"

Frank: "What, like with my Dad?"

HL: "Perhaps. What do you think?"

Frank: "He made me do horrible things."

HL: "Might the something up there be connected to the horrible things, do you think?"

Frank: "Well, yes, I felt so, I felt so . . . I don't know, I felt so . . ."

HL: "What angry? Cross, or . . . something else?"

Frank: Yes! [*With determination*] Angry with him."

Frank and I then go on to talk more about whether "angry" and "anger", for the time being, fit as terms for the "something up there". We explore the size of the "something up there", and as we carry on talking, Frank connects his self-hitting to his experiences of gross physical abuse during his adolescence at the hands of his father (which he told me about in previous sessions). In situations that commonly arise in our work, where there are obvious differences in power and status and where one person has a greater facility with words and concepts, there is a danger of the practitioner constructing, or calling into being, problems that the client did not have. For example, in the conversation with Frank there is a possibility that the practitioner determines that Frank has problems with anger and, consequently, prescribes "anger management". To guard against premature conclusions, we can be assisted by the systemic practices that invite us to enter the client's logic, that invite us to join their grammar and language, and that help us to pay close attention to feedback.

Relational knowing, or knowing with *others.* Many of us have also had experiences of meeting with people who, in individual sessions, have struggled to articulate themselves. Yet in sessions with significant others with whom they feel comfortable, they have been much more engaged, often surprising us with their knowledge and ability. In the Foreword to this book, Tom Andersen reminds us how people may show different levels of capacity in different contexts and with different people. Shotter (1993) has introduced the term "relational knowing" to distinguish between different types of knowledge. Factual knowledge, or the "knowing that" (e.g., that 2 and 2 is 4) is distinguished from a "knowing with"—a knowing that develops and emerges in interaction with others.

Slowing the pace. Denise Cardone and Amanda Hilton (chapter five) provide a beautiful example of the different and slower pace at which conversations may need to proceed in order to include everyone. As the example they present shows, they sit with silences and give Pete time to find and to speak his own words. Many people have commented (e.g., Goldberg et al., 1995; Fidell, 2000) that sessions can appear slowed down and that the therapeutic work may take longer. However, this may also have the advantages of giving time to listen in a new way and of not understanding too quickly. As the example with Pete shows, we should also remember that people with only a few words can say some important things.

Balancing the different voices. In order to avoid a difference that is too unusual (Andersen, 1992), it is important to respect an existing and established conversational pattern. By this we mean that while we always ensure that everyone has an opportunity to be heard in sessions, in families where other people always talk for the person with intellectual disabilities we do not try to "rescue" the situation by over-inviting the person with intellectual disabilities to speak (and thereby disqualifying or silencing others). In our experience it is a question of small steps and considered questions. One father (of a young man with severe intellectual disabilities) said to us: "It was not until I heard you asking for the third time, '*I wonder what John would say about that?*', that I had even considered that he could have an opinion about the things we were talking about."

Simplifying, repeating, and rephrasing language. Our language and sentences can often be complex and our pace too fast. At the same time, many people with intellectual disabilities work hard to be liked and accepted, or they may, like most people, not always wish to admit that they do not understand. Sometimes this process is referred to as acquiescing to, or agreeing with, anything that is suggested by a person who is in a more powerful position. Conversely, a person may use language or words that give the impression of a more sophisticated understanding than later turns out to be the case. Checking understanding frequently therefore becomes important, as does keeping a check of the differential levels of power that may be operating at any given time. As Fredman (chapter one) and Pote (chapter nine) point out, key to this task is the continued development of the practitioners' self-reflexivity and attention to ethical practices.

Abstractions and scaffolding. Many people with intellectual disabilities can be left behind by questions that are too abstract. For example, as one practitioner discovered, the question "How would you like support workers to be helpful to you?" was too abstract and complicated for Mary, who had a diagnosis of autism. Instead, a series of steps, drawing on the process that Vygotsky (1978) termed "scaffolding", proved helpful in enabling conversational participation. When the practitioner tried to establish Mary's answer to the above question, she used the following approach:

Practitioner: "Who works with you at home?"

Mary: "Suzanne."

Practitioner: "Anyone else?"

Mary: "And Donna."

Practitioner: "What do Suzanne and you do together?"

Mary: "We shop and do the bills."

Practitioner: "What do you like about the way Suzanne works with you?"

Mary: "She is good . . . she is kind . . . we have fun."

Practitioner: "Can you say some more?"

Mary: "Yes. She takes her time, she doesn't hurry, hurry."

Practitioner: "So let me see if I got that right. Suzanne doesn't hurry. She is kind. You have fun as well as doing work . . .?"

Mary: "Yes, and she comes every Tuesday . . . when she is not on holiday."

Gradually, and by breaking a question up into smaller units, a picture is built up of how Mary wants her support workers to help her. Such scaffolding practices can be used in numerous ways—for example, in inviting an "absent person" to join in the conversation: "I know Lisa isn't here with us now. I know this might seem a little strange. But I wonder if you can imagine her sitting here with us? In that blue chair. Can you touch the chair? Can you imagine Lisa there? What do you think she would say about . . . ?" We do, of course, recognize that there are many people for whom these practices are inaccessible. However, there have also been many people we have worked with who, over time have become accustomed to thinking about the ideas and views of others in their absence.

The concept of time. The concept of time and frequency can be bewildering for many people. For example, HL worked with a man who came to one session saying, "I haven't hit myself since I came last time [*four weeks previously*]. For ages. Since last Friday . . . Well, it is a least two months." Another person stated that something had happened a lot of times, "At least 50 times". A moment later she said, "No it was *more* than 50 times. It happened loads. It was at least 40 times." As Booth and Booth (1996) have pointed out, practitioners should be cautious in asking too many questions that are reliant on time and frequency responses, as this can cause unnecessary confusion or discomfort, especially if the exact timing is of little relevance to the work, or conversation, in hand. Providing linear chronological histories can also be difficult for many people. It can therefore often be more useful to think about a person's history as being a history of people rather than of chronological events.

Drawing, showing, and writing. There are several ways in which one can facilitate conversations and make things more concrete and accessible—for example, by drawing a picture of all the important people in someone's life, or of all the things that are going well; by showing or drawing the size of a worry/problem, which can often be easier to deal with in its externalized form; or by writing down and taking notes of important events. Fuchs, Mattison, and Sugden (2003) give an example of facilitating Peter, a man with intellectual disabilities, to understand his mother's stomach cancer, her treatment, and her subsequent recovery. Peter drew a picture of his mother, and he and the therapist drew the cancer onto the picture as his mother was talking about her illness and the operation. Using their drawing, the therapist and Peter "then cut the cancer out with scissors and replaced it with new paper which was described as 'healthy tissue'" (p. 21).

Photographs, video, and objects. Photographs of people and places can greatly enhance and facilitate conversations and understanding. We have met many people who may have difficulties in recalling or saying a person's name, but who join in conversations when photos are available. Speech and language therapists can often be immensely helpful in suggesting how we build and maintain conversational bridges. Video equipment may be used to record sessions. As Gaddis (2004) has shown in another context, watching video recordings of sessions with clients can create opportunities for new meanings to emerge and for further possibilities of change to open up. Finally, objects may be used in ways that open space for imagination and playful approaches to tackling concerns.

Pace of reflections. Cardone and Hilton (chapter five) recommend that when offering reflections, perhaps through a discussion by a reflecting team in the room, it is preferable to offer just a few comments and to start with reflections that refer to or include the person with intellectual disability. Prefacing a reflection or comment by clearly stating the name of the person for whom the comment is intended can also be helpful in (re)gaining a person's attention. Similarly, using the particular words or expressions that a person has used may foreground something that both makes the person attend and signals that they have been heard.

Practical arrangements. To facilitate participation, some people will require support with transport, buildings and rooms that are wheelchair-accessible, and reminders of appointments. The settings for sessions may also change according to people's circumstances. Baum and Walden (chapter four) describe an example where sessions switched to the family home when the father in the family became housebound due to illness. This, in turn, requires negotiation as to how sessions are conducted in a way that respects people's homes, minimizes interruptions, and ensures that the practitioners can work in ways that allow them to be most helpful to the family.

The use of metaphors and stories. Cardone and Hilton (chapter five) provide a number of examples where the person with intellectual disabilities brings a reference to a television programme or a metaphor to the session. They show how the elaboration and use of metaphors, "story-telling", and fictional characters can provide fertile material for enriching and engaging therapeutic conversations.

Who needs to be in conversation with whom about what? People with intellectual disabilities often have a lifelong dependency on others and may live within complex networks consisting of family, carers, and professionals. As they seldom initiate their own referrals, problems can readily be located within them without reference to the contributions of the wider system. It is good practice therefore, when receiving a referral, to consider who should be in conversations with whom about what. Many people will undoubtedly be familiar with situations where it has been by virtue of inviting referrers and significant members in a network to be in conversation with each other that the "problem" that was located in the person with intellectual disabilities, gets reframed, re-located, dis-solved, or transformed (see also Lang & McAdam, 1995). This is beautifully illustrated by Selma Rikberg Smyly with her example of "John" (chapter eight).

How can I show this is a useful model?

Readers of this volume, colleagues, and managers of practitioners who work systemically may have a number of questions about the effectiveness of systemic approaches in the field of intellectual disabilities—questions such as: *"Does it make a difference to people?" "What are the benefits?" "How does it compare to other therapeutic approaches?" "What do people with intellectual disabilities say about it?"* and so forth. These are important questions, and they are also of interest to many practitioners in the field. It is worth approaching these questions from a number of different angles, however.

First, it should be re-emphasized that the use of systemic approaches in working with people with intellectual disabilities has a relatively short history. So far, it has involved few practitioners working with a relatively small group of people and often in isolation from each other. Although reports in the literature point to the considerable opportunities offered by systemic approaches in working with people with intellectual disabilities, there is, as yet, no therapeutic process or outcome research (see Pote, chapter nine).

Second, there are a number of different ways of addressing the questions about the usefulness of a particular therapeutic approach, and the methods adopted will vary depending on what model or paradigm is employed. Within a modernist paradigm, randomized control trials are considered as the "gold standard" for investigating such questions. A number of large-scale studies have been conducted using this method to investigate the effectiveness of systemic therapy compared to other treatment approaches (Jones & Asen, 2000; Seikkula et al., 2003). Although these studies have not been concerned with people with intellectual disabilities, they have all shown evidence for the effectiveness of systemic therapy compared to other forms of interventions. Randomized controlled trials exploring the usefulness of systemic therapy with people with intellectual disabilities are, as yet, likely to be a distant vision. As Oliver et al. (2002) have observed, issues like capacity and consent may impede the development of such an evidence base, and, as has already been mentioned, the population of people with intellectual disabilities is small and the number of practitioners working systemically even smaller. However, this book and descriptions in the literature have shown that there are beginning to be descriptive accounts suggesting that systemic approaches offer opportunities to address the emotional and behavioural needs of clients with intellectual disabilities and the systems in which they live (see Halliday & Robbins, chapter three, and Pote, chapter nine). Moreover, using qualitative methods of investigation, there are, to our knowledge, three research studies that have sought to find answers to some of the questions posed. Thus, Arkless (2005) discovered a mixed range of views when she interviewed ten families who had been invited to participate in systemic family therapy. Some family members saw it as having a positive impact on their views about and ways of approaching difficulties they were facing. For other families, however, systemic therapy had not offered the kind of help they had expected, and the experience was seen as relatively insignificant or confusing. For the participants with intellectual disabilities, there was a general sense that the opportunity to talk about difficulties was seen as valuable. However, the degree to which some of these participants felt they had a voice again varied. A combination of feeling pressure to "know" what to say, and the presence of other family members in the meetings, had made it difficult for them to always have their say. This study has important implications for how practitioners explain and conduct their sessions. The other two studies are referred to in this book: Pote (2004) (see also chapter nine) investigated therapists' accounts of systemic family therapy with this client group, and Baum and Walden (chapter four) attempted to evaluate the effectiveness of their family therapy service in a community setting.

Third, it is important to bear in mind that although currently little therapeutic process or outcome research exists, it does not therefore follow that the approach is ineffectual. While it is our hope that this book will encourage practitioners to also consider undertaking research in this area, it can be challenging to conduct investigations using a modernist paradigm in the field of systemic therapy (Chase & Holmes, 1990; Sprenkle & Moon, 1996). Jennifer Clegg and Susan King (chapter seven) give an interesting example of how the outcome of a piece of family work could have been described either as a "failure" or as a "success" depending on when its impact was being "measured". Sprenkle and Moon (1996) have also pointed out that it is easier to measure change in individuals than in dyads or families, and therefore first-order change remains the most reliably used criterion.

Fourth, as we have already mentioned, there are different ways of conceptualizing research. One of the critiques of quantitative research is that it seems to take little account of views of science as a human endeavour and cultural practice (White, 1995). In many traditional quantitative studies, "the particularities of therapy outcomes, the local stories, cultural belonging and personal voices of participants have been 'smoothed' out of the text and subsumed into grand narratives about, for example, addiction, abuse or eating disorders" (Speedy, 2004, p. 44). It may be of interest to note that practitioners working within the narrative school and informed by postmodern theories conceive of the therapeutic conversations as "primary" research. For example, Epston (2001) argues:

> I have always thought of myself as doing research, but on problems and the relationships that people have with problems, rather than on the people themselves. The structuring of narrative questions

and interviews allows me and others to co-research problems and the alternative knowledges that are developed to address them. [Epston, 2001, p. 178; quoted in Dulwich Centre Publications, 2004, p. 30]

As Epston suggests, the practitioners and the people who come to consult them are seen as co-researchers "who are investigating the effects of problems and the client's solution knowledges" (Speedy, 2004, p. 44). These ways of conceiving of research and co-research have led to some interesting projects in which practitioners and their clients have built up archives of the therapy, the outcome, and the knowledge that has been gained from the therapy, with the aim of making these accounts and stories available to others facing similar difficulties. Archives can be built up in a number of different ways and using a number of different media:

> Archival documents can take the form of written documents, such as journal entries, letters, transcripts, or poems, or of visual depictions, such as paintings, drawings or collages. They can also take the form of audio taped or videotaped conversations. . . . Archival documents can be read aloud to people during therapy or they can be given to people to take home to peruse at their convenience. [Dulwich Centre Publications, 2004, p. 32]

We hope that readers will be inspired to consider a number of different ways of investigating the usefulness of systemic approaches. These may range from employing more conventional methodologies, involving multi-centre collaboration between practitioners, to small-scale research studies using both quantitative and qualitative approaches. But local knowledge can also be derived from producing single-outcome studies, where the people with intellectual disabilities and their systems are co-researchers. These stories could, as Speedy (2004) points out, form archives that could be shared with others and, over time, produce cumulative practice-based evidence of the experiences of working systemically with people affected with intellectual disabilities.

REFERENCES

American Association on Mental Retardation (2002). *Mental Retardation: Definitions, Classification and Systems of Supports* (10th edition). Washington, DC: American Association on Mental Retardation.

Andersen, T. (1987). The reflecting team: Dialogue and meta-dialogue in clinical work. *Family Process*, 26: 415–428.

Andersen, T. (1991). *The Reflecting Team: Dialogues and Dialogues about Dialogues.* New York: Norton.

Andersen, T. (1992). Reflections on reflecting with families. In: S. McNamee & K. Gergen (Eds.), *Therapy as Social Construction* (pp. 54–68). London: Sage.

Andersen, T. (1995). Reflecting processes: Acts of informing and forming. You can borrow my eyes, but you must not take them away from me! In: S. Friedman (Ed.), *The Reflecting Team in Action* (pp. 11–37). New York: Guilford Press.

Anderson, H. (1995). Collaborative language systems: Toward a post-modern therapy. In: R. Mikesell, D. Lusterman, & S. McDaniel (Eds.), *Integrating Family Therapy: Handbook of Family Psychology and Systems Theory* (pp. 27–44). Washington, DC: American Psychiatric Association.

Anderson, H., & Goolishian, H. (1986). Problem-determined systems—towards transformation in family therapy. *Journal of Strategic and Systemic Therapies*, 5: 1–13.

Anderson, H., & Goolishian, H. (1988). Human systems as linguistic system: Preliminary and evolving ideas about the implications for clinical theory. *Family Process*, 27: 371–393.

Anderson, H., & Goolishian, H. (1992). The client is the expert: A not-knowing approach to therapy. In: S. McNamee & K. J. Gergen (Eds.), *Therapy as Social Construction* (pp. 25–39). London: Sage.

Arkless, L. (2005). *Talking to People with Learning Disabilities and Their Families about the Experience of Systemic Therapy.* Doctoral Dissertation, University College London, London.

Arthur, A. R. (1999). Emotions and people with learning difficulty: Are clinical psychologists doing enough? *Clinical Psychology Forum*, 132: 39–43.

Atkinson, L., Chisholm, V., Scott, B., Goldberg, S., Vaughan, B., Blackwell, J.,

Dickens, S., & Tam, F. (1999). Maternal sensitivity, child functional level, and attachment in Down's syndrome. In: *Monographs of the Society for Research in Child Development, Vol. 64* (pp. 45–66). Oxford: Blackwell.

Bank-Mikkelsen, N. (1980). Denmark. In: R. Flynn & K. Nitsch (Eds.), *Normalisation, Social Integration and Community Services* (pp. 51–70). Austin, TX: Pro-Ed.

Barker, D. (1983). How to curb the fertility of the unfit: The feeble-minded in Edwardian Britain. *Oxford Journal of Education, 9* (3): 197–211.

Bateson, G. (1972). *Steps to an Ecology of Mind*. New York: Ballantine. Reprinted London: Paladin, 2000.

Baum, S., Chapman, K., Scior, K., Sheppard, N., & Walden, S. (2001). Themes emerging from systemic therapy involving adults with learning disabilities and their families. *Clinical Psychology, 3:* 16–18.

Beail, N. (1995). Outcome of psychoanalysis, psychoanalytic psychodynamic psychotherapy with people with intellectual disabilities: A review. *Changes, 13:* 186–191.

Beavers, J., Hampson, R. B., Hulgus, Y. F., & Beavers, W. R. (1986). Coping in families with a retarded child. *Family Process, 25:* 365–378.

Beavers, R., & Hampson, R. B. (2000). The Beavers systems model of family functioning. *Journal of Systemic Therapy, 2:* 128–143.

Beavers, W. R., & Hampson, R. B. (1990). *Successful Families: Assessment and Intervention*. New York: Norton.

Bender, M. (1993). The unoffered chair: The history of therapeutic disdain towards people with a learning difficulty. *Clinical Psychology Forum, 54:* 7–12.

Bennun, I. (1989). Perception of the therapist in family therapy. *Journal of Family Therapy, 11:* 243–255.

Benson, M. J., Schindler-Zimmerman, T., & Martin, D. (1991). Accessing children's perceptions of their family: Circular questioning revisited. *Journal of Marital and Family Therapy, 17, 4:* 363–372.

Berger, M. (1996). *Outcomes and Effectiveness in Clinical Practice*. Division of Clinical Psychology, Occasional Paper No. 1. Leicester: BPS.

Besa, D. (1994). Evaluating narrative family therapy using single-system research designs. *Research on Social Work Practice, 4* (3): 309–325.

Besley, T. (2001). Foucauldian influences in narrative therapy: An approach for school. *Journal of Educational Enquiry, 2* (2): 72–93.

Bicknell, J. (1983). The psychopathology of handicap. *British Journal of Medical Psychology, 56:* 161–178.

Blacher, J. (Ed.) (1984). *Severely Handicapped Children and Their Families: Research in Review*. New York: Academic Press.

Black, D. (1987). Handicap and family therapy. In: A. Bentovim, G. Gorell Barnes, & A. Cooklin (Eds.), *Family Therapy: Complementary Frameworks of Theory and Practice* (pp. 217–236). London: Academic Press.

Bloomfield, S., Nielsen, S., & Kaplan, L. (1984). Retarded adults, their families, and larger systems: A new role for the family therapist. *Family Therapy Collections, 11:* 138–149.

Booth, T., & Booth, W. (1996). Sounds of silence: Narrative research with inarticulate subjects. *Disability and Society, 11* (1): 55–69.
Boscolo, L., & Bertrando, P. (1996). *Systemic Therapy with Individuals*. London: Karnac.
Boscolo, L., Cecchin, G., Hoffman, L., & Penn, P. (1987). *Milan Systemic Therapy*. New York: Basic Books.
Boyle, B., Clancy, A., Connolly, A., Daly, E., Heffernan, B., Howley, E., Keena, M., McSharry, M., Moloney, G., Morrell, S., Murphy, C., Murphy, N., Murphy, T., Murtagh, M., Murray, L., Murray, P., Oulton, K. T., Richards, A., O'Riordan, J., Roche, D., Smyth, R., Tormey, A., & Walsh, P. (2003). The same in difference: The work of the peer counselors of the Irish wheelchair association and the national council of the blind of Ireland. *International Journal of Narrative Therapy and Community Work, 2*: 3–17.
Brent, D. A., Kolko, D., Birmaher, B., Baugher, M., Roth, C., Iyengar, S., & Johnson, B. A. (1997). A clinical psychotherapy trial for adolescent depression comparing cognitive, family and supportive therapy. *Archives of General Psychiatry, 54*: 887–895.
British Psychological Society (2001). *Learning Disability: Definitions and Contexts*. Leicester: BPS.
Bromley, J. (1998). Working with families. In: E. Emerson, C. Hatton, J. Bromley, & A. Caine (Eds.), *Clinical Psychology and People with Intellectual Disabilities* (pp. 247–264). Chichester: Wiley.
Brown, H., & Smith, H. (1989). "Whose ordinary life is it anyway?" *Disability, Handicap and Society, 4* (2): 105–119.
Brown, H., & Smith, H. (1992). Assertion, not assimilation: A feminist perspective on the normalisation principle. In: H. Brown & H. Smith (Eds.), *Normalisation: A Reader for the Nineties* (pp. 149–171). London: Routledge.
Burnham, J. (1992). Approach—Method—Technique: Making distinctions and creating connections. *Human Systems: Journal of Systemic Consultation & Management, 3*: 3–26.
Burr, V. (1995). *An Introduction to Social Constructionism*. London: Routledge.
Byng-Hall, J. (1995). *Rewriting Family Scripts*. London: Guilford Press.
Byrne, E. A., & Cunningham, C. C. (1985). The effects of mentally handicapped children on families—a conceptual review. *Journal of Child Psychology and Psychiatry, 26* (6): 847–864.
Caine, A., Hatton, C., & Emerson, E. (1998). Service provision. In: E. Emerson, C. Hatton, J. Bromley, & A. Caine (Eds.), *Clinical Psychology and People with Intellectual Disabilities* (pp. 54–75). Chichester: Wiley.
Campbell, D. (1995). *Learning Consultation: A Systemic Framework*. London: Karnac.
Campbell, D. (2000). *The Socially Constructed Organization*. London: Karnac.
Campbell, D. (2003). The mutiny and the bounty: The place of Milan ideas today. *Australian New Zealand Journal of Family Therapy, 24* (1): 15–25.
Campbell, D., Coldicott, T., & Kinsella, K. (1994). *Systemic Work with Organizations*. London: Karnac.

Campbell, D., Draper, R., & Crutchley, E. (1991). The Milan systemic approach to family therapy. In: A. Gurman & D. Kniskern (Eds.), *Handbook of Family Therapy*, 11 (pp. 325–362). New York: Brunner-Mazel.

Campbell, D., Draper, R., & Huffington, C. (1989). *Second Thoughts on the Theory and Practice of the Milan Approach*. London: Karnac.

Campbell, D., Draper, R., & Huffington, C. (1991). *A Systemic Approach to Consultation*. London: Karnac.

Carey, M., & Russell, S. (2003). Re-authoring: Some answers to commonly asked questions. *International Journal of Narrative Therapy and Community Work*, 3: 60–72.

Carr, A. (1991). Milan systemic therapy: A review of ten empirical investigations. *Journal of Family Therapy*, 13: 237–263.

Carr, A. (2000a). *Family Therapy: Concept, Process and Practice*. Chichester: Wiley.

Carr, A. (Ed.) (2000b). Special issue: Empirical approaches to family assessment. *Journal of Systemic Therapy*, 22 (2): 121–238.

Carter, B., & McGoldrick, M. (Eds.) (1989). *The Changing Family Life-Cycle: A Framework for Family Therapy* (2nd edition). Boston: Allyn & Bacon.

Cecchin, G. (1987). Hypothesizing, circularity and neutrality revisited: An invitation to curiosity. *Family Process*, 26: 405–413.

Cecchin, G. (1992). Constructing therapeutic possibilities. In: S. McNamee & K. J. Gergen (Eds.), *Therapy as Social Construction* (pp. 86–96). London: Sage.

Cecchin, G., Lane, G., & Ray, W. (1992). *Irreverence: A Strategy for Therapist Survival*. London: Karnac.

Cecchin, G., Lane, G., & Ray, W. (1994). *The Cybernetics of Prejudices in the Practice of Psychotherapy*. London: Karnac.

Chase, J., & Holmes, J. (1990). A two year audit of a systemic therapy clinic in adult psychiatry. *Journal of Systemic Therapy*, 12: 229–242.

Clare, D., & Grant, H. (1994). Sexual-abuse therapy and recovery group (STAR): A New Zealand program using narrative therapy for women survivors of childhood sexual abuse who are intellectually disabled. *Developmental Disabilities Bulletin*, 22 (2): 80–92.

Clegg, J. (1993). Putting people first: A social constructionist approach to learning difficulty. *British Journal of Clinical Psychology*, 3: 389–406.

Clegg, J. A. (2004). How can services become more ethical? In: W. R. Lindsay, J. L. Taylor, & P. Sturmey (Eds.), *Offenders with Developmental Disability* (pp. 91–108). Chichester: Wiley.

Clegg, J. A., & Lansdall-Welfare, R. (1995). Attachment and learning disability: A theoretical review informing three clinical interventions. *Journal of Intellectual Disability Research*, 39: 295–305.

Clegg, J. A., & Lansdall-Welfare, R. (2003). Death, disability and dogma. *Philosophy, Psychiatry and Psychology*, 10: 67–79.

Clegg, J. A., & Sheard, C. (2002). Challenging behaviour and insecure attachment. *Journal of Intellectual Disability Research*, 46: 503–506.

Clegg, J. A., Sheard, C., Cahill, J., & Osbeck, L. (2001). Severe learning disability and transition to adulthood. *British Journal of Medical Psychology, 74*: 151–166

Clements, J. (1987). *Severe Learning Difficulties and Psychological Handicap.* London: Wiley.

Clements, J. (1992). I can't explain ... "challenging behaviour": Towards a shared conceptual framework. *Clinical Psychology Forum, 39*: 29–37.

Cleveland, D., & Miller, N. (1977). Attitudes and family commitments of older siblings of mentally retarded adults: An exploratory study. *Mental Retardation, 15*: 38–41.

Cobb, H. C., & Gunn, W. (1994). Family interventions. In: D. C. Strohmer & H. T. Prout (Eds.), *Counselling and Psychotherapy with Persons with Mental Retardation and Borderline Intelligence* (pp. 235–255). Brandon, VT: Clinical Psychology Publishing.

Combs, G., & Freedman, J. (1998). Tellings and retellings. *Journal of Marital and Family Therapy, 24* (4): 405–408.

Craft, A. (1987). Mental handicap and sexuality: Issues for individuals with a mental handicap, their parents and professionals. In: A. Craft (Ed.), *Mental Handicap and Sexuality: Issues and Perspectives* (pp. 13–34). London: Costello.

Crnic, K. A., Friedrich, W. N., & Greenberg, M. T. (1983). Adaptation of families with mentally retarded children: A model of stress, coping and family ecology. *American Journal of Mental Deficiency, 88*: 125–138.

Cronen, V. E. (1994). Co-ordinated management of meaning: Practical theory for the complexities and contradictions of everyday life. In: J. Siegfried (Ed.), *The Status of Common Sense in Psychology* (pp. 125–139). Norwood, NJ: Ablex.

Cronen, V., & Lang, P. (1994). Language and action: Wittgenstein and Dewey in the practice of therapy and consultation. *Human Systems: Journal of Systemic Consultation and Management, 5*: 5–43.

Cronen, V., & Pearce, B. W. (1985). Toward an explanation of how the Milan method works: An invitation to a systemic epistemology and the evolution of family systems. In D. Campbell & R. Draper, *Applications of Systemic Family Therapy: The Milan Approach* (pp. 69–84). London: Grune & Stratton.

Cummins, R. (1991). Comprehensive Quality of Life Scale—Intellectual Disability: An instrument under development. *Australia and New Zealand Journal of Developmental Disabilities, 17* (2): 259-64.

Cummins, R. (2001). The subjective well-being of people caring for a family member with a severe disability at home: A review. *Journal of Intellectual and Developmental Disability, 26*: 83–100.

Cummins, R. (2004). "Service Providers as Managers of Clients' Subjective Well-Being." Keynote address to Towards Mutual Understanding, 12th IASSID World Congress, Montpellier.

Dagnan, D., & Ruddick, L. (1995). The use of analogue scales and personal questionnaires for interviewing people with learning disabilities. *Clinical Psychology Forum, 79*: 21–24.

Dale, N. (1995). *Working with Families of Children with Special Needs: Partnership and Practice.* London: Routledge.
Dallos, R., & Draper, R. (2000). *An Introduction to Family Therapy: Systemic Theory and Practice.* Buckingham: Open University Press.
Danforth, S., & Navaro, V. (1998). Speech acts: Sampling the social construction of mental retardation in everyday life. *Mental Retardation, 36:* 31–43.
Davidson, J., Lax. W., & Lussardi, D. J. (1990). Use of the reflecting team in the initial interview and in supervision and training. In: T. Andersen (Ed.), *The Reflecting Team* (pp. 134–156). New York: Norton.
Davies, C. A., & Jenkins, R. (1997). "She has different fits to me": How people with learning difficulties see themselves. *Disability and Society, 12:* 95–109.
Department of Health (1992). *Social Care for Adults with Learning Disabilities (Mental Handicap),* LAC (92) 15. London: HMSO.
Department of Health (1999). *National Service Framework for Mental Health.* London: HMSO.
Department of Health (2001). *Valuing People: A New Strategy for Learning Disability for the 21st Century.* London: HMSO.
Department of Health (2002). *Valuing People: Towards Person Centred Approaches.* London: HMSO.
Department of Health & Social Security (1971). *Better Services for the Mentally Handicapped.* Cmnd 4683. London: HMSO.
de Shazer, S. (1985). *Keys to Solution in Brief Therapy.* London: Norton.
de Shazer, S. (1988). *Clues: Investigating Solutions in Brief Therapy.* London: Norton.
Dixon, M., & Matthews, S. (1992). Learning difficulty in the family: Making systemic approaches relevant. *Clinical Psychology Forum, 39:* 17–21.
Donati, S., Glynn, B., Lynggaard, H., & Pearce, P. (2000). Systemic interventions in a learning disability service: An invitation to join. *Clinical Psychology Forum, 144:* 24–27.
Dowling, M., & Dolan, L. (2001). Families with children with disabilities: Inequalities and the social model. *Disability and Society, 16* (1): 21–35.
Drotar, D. D., & Sturm, L. A. (1996). Interdisciplinary collaboration in the practice of mental retardation. In: J. W. Jacobson & J. A. Mulick (Eds.), *Manual of Diagnosis and Professional Practice in Mental Retardation* (pp. 393–401). Washington, DC: American Psychological Association.
Dulwich Centre Publications (2004). Narrative therapy and research. *International Journal of Narrative Therapy and Community Work, 2:* 29–36.
Ekdawi, I., Gibbons, S., Bennett, E., & Hughes, G. (2000). *Whose Reality Is It Anyway? Putting Social Constructionist Philosophy into Everyday Practice.* Brighton: Pavilion.
Elizur, Y. (1993). Ecosystemic training: Conjoining supervision and organisational development. *Family Process, 32:* 185–201.
Elliot, R. (1989). Comprehensive process analysis: Understanding the change process in significant therapy events. In: M. J. Packer & R. B. Addison (Eds.),

Entering the Circle: Hermeneutic Investigation in Psychology (pp.165–184). Albany, NY: SUNY Press.

Epston, D. (1999). Co-research: The making of an alternative knowledge. In: *Narrative Therapy and Community Work: A Conference Collection* (pp. 137–158). Adelaide: Dulwich Centre Publications.

Epston, D. (2001). Anthropology, archives, co-research and narrative therapy. In: D. Denborough (Ed.), *Family Therapy: Exploring the Field's Past, Present and Possible Futures* (pp. 177–182). Adelaide: Dulwich Centre Publications.

Epston, D., White, M., & Murray, K. (1992). A proposal for a re-authoring therapy: Rose's revisioning of her life and a commentary. In: S. McNamee & K. Gergen (Eds.), *Therapy as Social Construction* (pp. 96–115). London: Sage.

Evans, A., & Midence, K. (1999). Is there a role for family therapy in adults with a learning difficulty? *Clinical Psychology Forum, 29*: 30–34.

Evans, K., & Carter, C. O. (1954). Care and disposal of mongolian defectives. *Lancet, 2*: 960–963.

Fatimilehin, I. A., & Nadirshaw, Z. (1994). A cross-cultural study of parental attitudes and beliefs about learning disability (mental handicap). *Mental Handicap Research, 7* (3): 202–227.

Fernald, W. E. (1893). The history of the treatment of the feeble-minded. In: *Report of the Proceedings of the 20th National Conference of Charities and Correction*. Boston: G. H. Ellis.

Ferns, P. (1992). Promoting race equality through normalisation. In: H. Brown & H. Smith (Eds.), *Normalisation: A Reader for the Nineties* (pp. 134–147). London: Routledge.

Fidell, B. (1996). Making family therapy user-friendly for learning disabled clients. *Context, 26*: 11–13.

Fidell, B. (2000). Exploring the use of family therapy with adults with a learning disability. *Journal of Family Therapy, 22*: 308–323.

Finlay, M., & Lyons, E. (1998). Social identity and people with learning difficulties: Implications for self-advocacy groups. *Disability and Society, 13*: 37–51.

Flaskas, C. (2000). "An Argument for Theory Diversity in Family Therapy." Paper presented at the 12th IFTA Family Therapy World Congress, Oslo.

Flaskas, C., & Perlesz, A. (Eds.) (1996). *The Therapeutic Relationship in Systemic Therapy*. London: Karnac.

Folkman, S., Schaefer, C., & Lazarus, R. S. (1979). Cognitive processes as mediators of stress and coping. In: V. Hamilton & D. W Warburton (Eds.), *Human Stress and Cognition* (pp. 265–298). New York: Wiley.

Foster, M. (1988). A systems perspective and families of handicapped children. *Journal of Family Psychology, 2*: 54–56.

Foucault, M. (1980). *Power/Knowledge: Selected Interviews and Other Writings*. New York: Pantheon Books.

Fox, H. (2003). Using therapeutic documents: A review. *International Journal of Narrative Therapy and Community Work. 4*: 26–37.

Fox, H., Tench, C., & Marie (2002). Outsider-witness practices and group supervision. *International Journal of Narrative Therapy and Community Work*, 4: 25–32.
Fredman, G. (1997). *Death Talk: Conversations with Children and Families*. London: Karnac.
Fredman, G. (2001). Editorial. Systemic practice with clinical psychology: Why not? *Clinical Psychology*, 3: 4–7.
Fredman, G. (2004). *Transforming Emotion: Conversations in Counselling and Psychotherapy*. London: Whurr.
Fredman, G., & Dalal, G. (1998). Ending discourses: Implications for relationships and action in therapy. *Human Systems*, 9 (1): 1–13.
Freedman, J., & Combs, C. (1996). *Narrative Therapy: The Social Construction of Preferred Realities*. New York: Norton.
Freeman, J., Epston, D., & Lobovits, D. (1997). *Playful Approaches to Serious Problems: Narrative Therapy with Children and Their Families*. New York: Norton.
Fruggeri, L. (1992). Therapeutic process as the social construction of change. In: S. McNamee & K. J. Gergen (Eds.), *Therapy as Social Construction* (pp. 40–53). London: Sage.
Fryers, T. (1993). Epidemiological thinking in mental retardation: Issues in taxonomy and population frequency. In: N. W. Bray (Ed.), *International Review of Research in Mental Retardation, Vol. 19* (pp. 97–133). San Diego, CA: Academic Press.
Fuchs, K., Mattison, V., & Sugden, C. (2003). Reflections on engagement. *Context*, 65: 21–22.
Furlong, M., Young, J., Perlesz, A., McLachlan, D., & Reiss, C. (1991). For family therapists involved in the treatment of chronic and longer-term conditions. *Dulwich Centre Newsletter*, 4: 58–68.
Gaddis, S. (2004). Repositioning traditional research: Centring clients' accounts in the construction of professional therapy knowledges. *International Journal of Narrative Therapy and Community Work*, 2: 37–48.
Gallagher, E. (2002). Adult clients with mild "intellectual disability": Rethinking our assumptions. *Australian and New Zealand Journal of Family Therapy*, 23 (4): 202–210.
Gangadharan, S., Bretherton, K., & Johnson, B. (2001). Pattern of referral to a child learning disability service. *British Journal of Developmental Disabilities*, 47 (93, Part 2): 99–104.
Gardner, A., & Rikberg Smyly, S. (1997). How do we stop "doing" and start listening: Responding to the emotional needs of people with learning disabilities. *British Journal of Learning Disabilities*, 25: 26–30.
Gath, A. (1973). The school age siblings of mongol children. *British Journal of Psychiatry*, 130: 405–410.
Gath, A., & Gumley, D. (1987). Retarded children and their siblings. *Journal of Child Psychology and Psychiatry*, 28: 715–730.
George, E., Iveson, C., & Ratner, H. (1990). *Problem to Solutions: Brief Therapy with Individuals and Families*. London: B.T. Press.

Gergen, K. J. (1994). *Realities and Relationships: Soundings in Social Construction*. Cambridge, MA: Harvard University Press.

Ghaziuddin, M. (1988). Behaviour disorders in the mentally handicapped: The role of life events. *British Journal of Psychiatry, 152*: 683–686.

Gleeson, B. (2003). "After Deinstitutionalisation: Do We Still Care?" Keynote address to Imagination & Innovation, 38th National Conference of ASSID, Brisbane.

Goldberg, D., Magrill, L., Hale, J., Damaskindou, K., Paul, J., & Tham, S. (1995). Protection and loss: Working with learning disabled adults and their families. *Journal of Family Therapy, 17*: 263–280.

Goldner, V. (1998). The treatment of violence and victimization in intimate relationships. *Family Process, 37*: 263–286.

Gorell Barnes, G., & Dowling, E. (2000). *Children, Parents and Divorce*. Basingstoke: Macmillan.

Gorell Barnes, G., Thompson, P., Daniel, G., & Burchardt, N. (1998). *Growing Up in Stepfamilies*. Oxford: Clarendon Press.

Grant, G. (1990). Elderly parents with handicapped children: Anticipating the future. *Journal of Aging Studies, 4* (4): 359–374.

Grant, G., & McGrath, M. (1990). Need for respite-care services for care-givers of persons with mental retardation. *American Journal of Mental Retardation, 94* (6): 638–648.

Greenberg, J. S., Seltzer, M. M., & Greenley, J. R. (1993). Aging parents of adults with disabilities: The gratifications and frustrations of later-life care giving. *Gerontologist, 33*: 542–550.

Griffith, J. L., & Elliott Griffith, M. (1994). *The Body Speaks: Therapeutic Dialogue for Mind–Body Problems*. New York: Basic Books.

Hailstone, E. (1997). *Family Psychology and Therapy Service: Family Satisfaction Study*. Report completed in part fulfilment of Doctorate in Clinical Psychology, University of Leeds.

Haley, J. (1975). Why a Mental Health Clinic should avoid family therapy. *Journal of Marriage and Family Counselling* (January): 3–13.

Hanley-Maxwell, C., Whitney-Thomas, J., & Pogoloff, S. (1995). The second shock. *Journal of the Association for Persons with Severe Handicaps, 20*: 3–15.

Hannah, C. (1994). The context of culture in systemic therapy: An application of CMM. *Human Systems, 5*: 29–81.

Hastings, R. P., Sonuga-Barke, J. S., & Remington, B. (1996). An analysis of labels for people with learning disabilities. *British Journal of Clinical Psychology, 32*: 463–465.

Hennicke, K. (1993). Systems therapy for persons with mental retardation. In: R. J. Fletcher & A. Dosen (Eds.), *Mental Health Aspects of Mental Retardation: Progress in Assessment and Treatment* (pp. 402–417). New York: Lexington.

Heslop, P., Mallett, R., Simons, K., & Ward, L. (2002). *Bridging the Divide at the Transition*. Kidderminster: BILD.

Hill, J., Fonagy, P., Safier, E., & Sargent, J. (2003). The ecology of attachment in the family. *Family Process, 42*: 205–221.

Hoffman, L. (1985). Beyond power and control: Toward a "second order" family systems therapy. *Family Systems Medicine, 3* (4): 381–396.
Hoffman, L. (1988). A constructivist position for family therapy. *The Irish Journal of Psychology, 9* (1): 110–129.
Hoffman, L. (1990). Constructing realities: An art of lenses. *Family Process, 29* (1): 1–13.
Hoffman, L. (1993). *Exchanging Voices: A Collaborative Approach to Family Therapy.* London: Karnac.
Holborn, S., & Vietze, P. (1998). Has person-centred planning become the alchemy of developmental disabilities? *Mental Retardation, 36*: 485–488.
Hollins, S., & Grimer, M. (1988). *Going Somewhere.* London: SPCK.
Hoper, J. H. (1999). Families who unilaterally discontinue narrative therapy: Their story, a qualitative study. *Dissertation Abstracts International: Section B: Sciences & Engineering, 60* (6): 29–45.
Houghton, B. (1999). *Audit of Referrals and Take-up of Service.* Report completed in part fulfilment of Doctorate in Clinical Psychology, University of Leeds.
Howe, R., & von Foerster, H. (1974). Cybernetics at Illinois. *Forum, 6*: 15–17.
Hubert, J. (1991). *Homebound: Crisis in the Care of Young People with Severe Learning Difficulties.* London: King's Fund.
Huffington, C., & Brunning, H. (1994). *Internal Consultancy in the Public Sector.* London: Karnac.
Huxley, A. (1932). *Texts and Pretexts: An Anthology with Commentaries.* London: Chatto & Windus.
Imber-Black, E. (1987). The mentally handicapped in context. *Family Systems Medicine, 5*: 428–445.
Imber-Black, E. (1988). *Families and Larger Systems: A Family Therapist's Guide Through the Labyrinth.* New York: Guilford Press
Ingram, J. (2000). *An Introduction to the Leeds FPTS: A Guide for People Joining the Team.* Leeds: Community and Mental Health NHS Teaching Trust.
Iveson, C. (1990). *Whose Life? Community Care of Older People and Their Families.* London: BT Press.
Jackson, M. (1996). Institutional provision for the feeble-minded in Edwardian England: Sandlebridge and the scientific morality of permanent care. In: D. Wright & A. Digby (Eds.), *From Idiocy to Mental Deficiency: Historical Perspectives on People with Learning Disabilities* (pp. 161–183). London: Routledge.
Janssen, C., Schuengel, C., & Stolk, J. (2002). Understanding challenging behaviour in people with severe and profound intellectual disability: A stress-attachment model. *Journal of Intellectual Disability Research, 46*: 445–453.
Jay, D. (1979). *Report of the Committee of Enquiry into Mental Handicap Nursing and Care.* Cmnd 746811. London: HMSO.
Jones, E., & Asen, E. (2000). *Systemic Couple Therapy and Depression.* London: Karnac.
Kazak, A. E., & Martin, R. S. (1984). Differences, difficulties and adaptation: Stress and social networks in families with a handicapped child. *Family Relations, 33*: 67–77.

Kensington Consultation Centre (2004). *What Does Systemic Mean?* Retrieved 22 November <http://www.kcc-international.com/courses/the_scho.htm>.

Kew, S. (1975). *Handicap and Family Crisis.* London: Pitman.

Kingston, P., & Smith, D. (1985). Live consultation without a one-way screen. *Australian and New Zealand Journal of Family Therapy, 6* (2): 71–75.

Lancioni, G. E., O'Reilly, M. F., & Emerson, E. (1996). A review of choice research with people with severe and profound developmental disabilities. *Research in Developmental Disabilities, 17* (5): 391–411.

Lang, P., & McAdam, E. (1995). Stories, giving accounts and systemic descriptions. Perspectives and positions in conversations. Feeding and fanning the winds of creative imagination. *Human Systems: Journal of Systemic Consultation and Management, 6:* 71–103.

Larner, G. (2004). Family therapy and the politics of evidence. *Journal of Family Therapy, 26:* 17–39.

La Vigna, G. W., & Donnellan, A. M. (1986). *Alternatives to Punishment: Solving Behavior Problems with Non-Aversive Strategies.* New York: Irvington.

Lax, W. (1995). Offering reflections: Some theoretical and practical considerations. In S. Friedman (Ed.), *The Reflecting Team in Action* (pp. 145–166). New York: Guildford Press.

Learning Disability Advisory Group (2001). *Fulfilling the Promises: Proposal for a Framework for Services for People with Learning Disability.* Cardiff: National Assembly for Wales.

Leeds FPTS (2002). *The Family Psychology and Therapy Service: Progress Review and Business Plan.* Leeds: Community and Mental Health Services NHS Teaching Trust.

Lindsay, W., Neilson, C., & Lawrence, H. (1997). Cognitive behaviour therapy for anxiety in people with learning disabilities. In: B. Kroese, D. Dagnan, & K. Loumidis (Eds.), *Cognitive-Behaviour Therapy for People with Learning Disabilities* (pp. 124–140). London: Routledge.

Lowe, E., & Guy, G. (1996). A reflecting team format for solution-oriented supervision: Practical guidelines and theoretical distinctions. *Journal of Systemic Therapies, 15* (4): 26–45.

Lynggaard, H., Donati, S., Pearce, P., & Sklavounos, D. (2001). A difference that made a difference: Introducing systemic ideas and practices into a multi-disciplinary learning disability service. *Clinical Psychology, 3:* 12-15.

Lynggaard, H., & Scior, K. (2002). Narrative therapy and people with learning disabilities. *Clinical Psychology, 17:* 33–36.

Madsen, W. C. (1999). *Collaborative Therapy with Multi-Stressed Families.* New York: Guilford Press.

Mason, B. (1991). *Handing Over: Developing Consistency across Shifts in Residential and Health Settings.* London: Karnac.

Matthews, B., & Gates, R. (2003). Finding new hearts on a journey through grief. In: I. Brown & R. I. Brown (Eds.), *Quality of Life and Disability: An Approach for Community Practitioners* (pp. 197–206). London: Jessica Kingsley.

Matthews, B., & Matthews, B., (2005). Narrative therapy: Potential uses for

people with intellectual disability. *International Journal of Disability, Community and Rehabilitation*, 4 (1).
Maturana, H. (1988). The search for objectivity or the quest for a compelling argument. *Irish Journal of Psychology*, 9: 25–82.
McCarthy, J., & Boyd, J. (2002). Mental health services and young people with intellectual disability: Is it time to do better? *Journal of Intellectual Disability Research*, 46 (3): 250–256.
McCarthy, M. (1999). *Sexuality and Women with Learning Disabilities*. London: Jessica Kingsley.
McConachie, H. (1993). Implications of a model of stress and coping for services to families of young disabled children. *Child Care, Health and Development*, 20: 37–46.
McIntosh, P. (2002). An archi-texture of learning disability services: The use of Michel Foucault. *Disability and Society*, 17 (1): 65–79.
McNamee, S., & Gergen, K. (1992). *Therapy as Social Construction*. Newbury Park, CA: Sage.
Mental Health Foundation (1996). *Building Expectations: Opportunities and Services for People with a Learning Disability. Report of the Mental Health Foundation Committee of Enquiry*. London: Mental Health Foundation.
Minuchin, S. (1974). *Families and Systemic Therapy*. London: Tavistock.
Minuchin, S. (1998). Where is the family in narrative family therapy? *Journal of Marital and Family Therapy*, 24 (4): 397–403.
Minuchin, S., & Fishman, H. C. (1981). *Family Therapy Techniques*. Cambridge, MA: Harvard University Press.
Mitchell, W., & Sloper, P. (2000). *User-Friendly Information for Families with Disabled Children: A Guide to Good Practice*. York: Joseph Rowntree Foundation.
Mittler, P., & Sinason, V. (Eds.) (1996). *Changing Policy and Practice for People with Learning Disabilities*. London: Cassell Education.
Morgan, A. (1997). Conversations of ability. *Dulwich Centre Newsletter*, 4: 12–19.
Morgan, A. (1998). Conversations of ability. In: C. White & D. Denborough (Eds.), *Introducing Narrative Therapy: A Collection of Practice Based Writing* (pp. 33–46). Adelaide: Dulwich Centre Publications.
Morgan, A. (Ed.) (1999). *Once Upon a Time . . . Narrative Therapy with Children and Their Families*. Adelaide: Dulwich Centre Publications.
Morgan, A. (2000). *What Is Narrative Therapy? An Easy-to-Read Introduction*. Adelaide: Dulwich Centre Publications.
Morgan, A. (2002). Beginning to use a narrative approach in therapy. *Clinical Psychology*, 17: 37–42.
Nirje, B. (1980). The normalisation principle. In: R. Flynn & K. Nitsch (Eds.), *Normalisation, Social Integration and Community Services* (pp. 31–50). Austin, TX: Pro-Ed.
O'Brien, J. (1987). A guide to life-style planning. In: G. T. Bellamy & B. Wilcox (Eds.), *A Comprehensive Guide to the Activities Catalogue: An Alternative Cur-*

riculum for Youths and Adults with Severe Disabilities (pp. 175–188). Baltimore, MD: Paul H. Brookes.

Oliver, P. C., Piachaud, J., Done, J., Regan, A., Cooray, S., & Tyrer, P. (2002). Difficulties in conducting a randomised controlled trial of health service interventions in intellectual disability: Implications for evidence-based practice. *Journal of Intellectual Disability Research*, 46 (4): 340–345.

Owens, R. J., & Ashcroft, J. B. (1982). Functional analysis in applied psychology. *British Journal of Clinical Psychology*, 21: 181–189.

Partridge, K., Bennett, E., Webster, A., & Ekdawi, I. (1995). Consultation with clients: An alternative way of working in adult mental health. *Clinical Psychology Forum*, 83: 26–28.

Pascall, G., & Hendy, N. (2004). Disability and transition to adulthood: The politics of parenting. *Critical Social Policy*, 24: 165–186.

People First (1995). *Central England People First: Aims*. Retrieved 5 December <http://www.peoplefirst.org.uk/aims.html>.

Percy, I. (1999). Sharon, the worry-lion tamer. In: A. Morgan (Ed.), *Once Upon a Time . . . Narrative Therapy with Children and Their Families*. Adelaide: Dulwich Centre Publications.

Perlesz, A., Young, J., Paterson, S., & Bridge, S. (1994). The reflecting team as a reflection of second order therapeutic ideals. *Australian and New Zealand Journal of Family Therapy*, 15 (3): 117–127.

Perry, L., & Gentle, S. J. (1997). Sarah-Jane's story. *Dulwich Centre Newsletter*, 4: 22–26.

Pote, H. (2001). A social constructionist approach in working with people with learning difficulties: Opportunities and constraints. *Psychology Research*, 10 (2): 49–71.

Pote, H. (2002). *Therapists' Accounts of Process of Systemic Family Therapy with People with Learning Disabilities and Their Families*. Doctoral dissertation, Salomons, Canterbury Christ Church University College, Tunbridge Wells.

Pote, H. (2004). Therapists' accounts of systemic family therapy with people with intellectual disabilities. *Journal of Intellectual Disability Research*, 48: 510–517.

Pote, H., King, S. J., & Clegg, J. A. (2004). Vulnerability, protection and blame in therapeutic conversations with families. *Journal of Intellectual Disability Research*, 48: 377.

Pote, H., Stratton, P., Cottrell, D., Shapiro, D., & Boston, P. (2003). Systemic family therapy can be manualized: Research process and findings. *Journal of Family Therapy*, 25: 236–262.

Potts, M., & Howard, A. (1986). Psychology and community mental handicap. In: H. Koch (Ed.), *Community Clinical Psychology* (pp. 46–84). London: Croom Helm.

Quarry, A., & Burbach, F. R. (1998). Clinical consultancy in adult mental health, integrating whole team training and supervision. *Clinical Psychology Forum*, 120: 14–17.

Race, D. (1995). Classification of people with learning disabilities. In: N. Malin (Ed.), *Services for People with Learning Disabilities* (pp. 13–29). London: Routledge.

Rapley, M., Kieman, P., & Antaki, C. (1998). Invisible to themselves or negotiating identity? The interactional management of "being intellectually disabled". *Disability and Society*, 13: 807–827.

Raval, H. (1996). A systemic perspective on working with interpreters. *Clinical Child Psychology and Psychiatry*, 1 (1): 29–43.

Raval, H. (2003). An overview of the issues in the work with interpreters. In: R. Tribe & H. Raval (Eds.), *Working with Interpreters* (pp. 8–29). Hove: Brunner-Routledge.

Real, T. (1990). The therapeutic use of self in constructionist/systemic therapy. *Family Process*, 29: 255–272.

Reder, P., & Fredman, G. (1996). The relationship to help: Interacting beliefs about the treatment process. *Clinical Child Psychology and Psychiatry*, 1 (3): 457–467.

Reinders, H. S. (2000). *The Future of the Disabled in Liberal Society: An Ethical Analysis*. Notre Dame, IN: Notre Dame Press.

Rhodes, J. (2000). Solution-focused consultation in a residential setting. *Clinical Psychology Forum*, 141: 29–33.

Rhodes, P. (2002). Mainstreaming intellectual disability into the history of family therapy. *Australian and New Zealand Journal of Family Therapy*, 23 (4): 211–214.

Rhodes, P. (2003). Behavioural and family systems interventions in developmental disability: Towards a contemporary and integrative approach. *Journal of Intellectual and Developmental Disability*, 28 (1): 51–64.

Risley, T. R., & Reid, D. H. (1996). Management and organisational issues in the delivery of psychological services for people with mental retardation. In: J. W. Jacobson & J. A. Mulick (Eds.), *Manual of Diagnosis and Professional Practice in Mental Retardation* (pp. 383–391). Washington, DC: APA.

Roccoforte, J. A. (1991). *Stress, Financial Burden and Coping Resources in Families Providing Home Care for Adults with Learning Disabilities*. Master's thesis, University of Illinois at Chicago.

Rose, N. (1999). *Governing the Soul: The Shaping of the Private Self* (2nd edition). London: Free Association Books.

Roth, A., & Fonagy, P. (1996). *What Works for Whom? A Critical Review of Psychotherapy Research*. New York: Guilford Press.

Roth, S., & Epston, D. (1995). *Framework for a White/Epston Type Interview*. Retrieved 5 December <http://www.narrativeapproaches.com/narrative%20 papers%20folder/white_interview.htm>.

Roy-Chowdhury, S. (1992). Family therapy, multidisciplinary teams and people with learning difficulties: A conversation. *Clinical Psychology Forum*, 39: 12–16.

Seikkula, J., Alakare, B., Aaltonen, J., Holma, J., Rasinkangas, A., & Lehtinen,

V. (2003). Open dialogue approach: Treatment principles and preliminary results of a two-year follow-up on first episode schizophrenia. *Ethical and Human Sciences and Service, 5* (3): 163–182.

Ryan, J., & Thomas, F. (1980). *The Politics of Mental Handicap.* London: Penguin.

Ryan, R. (1994). Post-traumatic stress disorder in persons with developmental disabilities. *Community Mental Health Journal, 30*: 45–54.

Sabat, S. R. (2001). *The Experience of Alzheimer's Disease: Life through a Tangled Veil.* Oxford: Blackwell.

Saetersdal, B. (1997). Forbidden suffering: The Pollyanna syndrome of the disabled and their families. *Family Process, 36*: 431–435.

Salmon, A. (1996). Family therapy and learning difficulties: A case discussion. *Context, 29*: 42–45.

Scottish Executive (2000). *The Same as You? A Review of Services for People with Learning Disabilities.* Edinburgh: Scottish Executive.

Seligman, M., & Darling, R. B. (1989). *Ordinary Families, Special Children: A Systems Approach to Childhood Disability.* New York: Guildford Press.

Seltzer, M. M. (1992). Family care giving across the full life span. In: L. Rowitz (Ed.), *Mental Retardation in the Year 2000* (pp. 85–99). London: Springer-Verlag.

Seltzer, M. M., & Krauss, M. W. (1989). Aging parents with adult mentally retarded children: Family risk factors and sources of support. *American Journal of Mental Retardation, 94* (3): 303–312.

Selvini Palazzoli, M. S., Boscolo, L., Cecchin, G., & Prata, G. (1980). Hypothesizing—circularity—neutrality: Three guidelines for the conductor of the session. *Family Process, 19*: 3–12.

Shotter, J. (1993). *Conversational Realities: Constructing Life through Language.* London: Sage.

Shulman, S. (1988). The family of the severely handicapped child: The sibling perspective. *Journal of Family Therapy, 10*: 125–134.

Silver, E. (1991). Should I give advice? A systemic view. *Journal of Family Therapy, 13*: 295–309.

Simons, K. (1992). *Sticking Up for Yourself: Self Advocacy and People with Learning Disabilities.* York: Joseph Rowntree Foundation.

Sinason, V. (1992). *Mental Handicap and the Human Condition: New Approaches from the Tavistock.* London: Free Association Books.

Skelly, A. (2002). Valuing People: A critical psychoanalytic perspective in reply to Baum and Webb. *Clinical Psychology, 18*: 42–45.

Sloper, P. (1999). Models of service support for parents of disabled children. What do we know? What do we need to know? *Child Care Health and Development, 25* (2): 85–99.

Smith, J., Jarman, M., & Osborn, M. (1999). Doing interpretative phenomenological analysis. In: M. Murray & K. Chamberlain (Eds.), *Qualitative Health Psychology: Theories and Methods* (pp. 218–240). London: Sage.

Snyder, W., & McCollum, E. (1999). Their home is their castle: Learning to do in-home systemic therapy. *Family Process, 38* (2): 229–242.

Speedy, J. (2004). Living a more peopled life: Definitional ceremony as inquiry into psychotherapy "outcomes". *International Journal of Narrative Therapy and Community Work, 3*: 43–53.

Sprague, S. (2000). The treatment effect of initial session unique outcome mindfulness in narrative therapy: An exploratory study. *Dissertation Abstracts International. Section B: Sciences and Engineering, 61* (4): 22–23.

Sprenkle, D. H., & Moon, S. M. (1996). *Research Methods in Systemic Therapy*. New York: Guilford Press.

Stack, L. S., Haldipur, C. V., & Thompson, H. (1987). Stressful life events and psychiatric hospitalization of mentally retarded patients. *American Journal of Psychiatry, 144*: 611–613.

Stenfert Kroese, B. (1997). Cognitive-behaviour therapy for people with learning disabilities: Conceptual and contextual issues. In: B. Stenfert Kroese, D. Dagnan, & K. Loumidis (Eds.), *Cognitive-Behaviour Therapy for People with Learning Disabilities* (pp. 1–15). London: Routledge.

Stenfert Kroese, B., Dagnan, D., & Loumidis, K. (Eds.) (1997). *Cognitive-Behaviour Therapy for People with Learning Disabilities*. London: Routledge.

St James-O'Connor, T., Meakes, E., Pickering, M. R., & Schuman, M. (1997). On the right track: Client experience of narrative therapy. *Contemporary Family Therapy, 19* (4): 479–495.

Stolk, J., & Kars, H. (2000). Parents' experiences of meaning. In: J. Stolk, T. Boer, & R. Seldenrijk (Eds.), *Meaningful Care: A Multidisciplinary Approach to the Meaning of Care for People with Mental Retardation* (pp. 11–38). London: Kluwer.

Street, E., & Downey, J. (1996). *Brief Therapeutic Consultations: An Approach to Systemic Counselling*. Chichester: Wiley.

Thomas, B. (2001). "I've taught you once already": Forgetting the disability in learning disability. *Clinical Psychology Forum, 148*: 26–28.

Thomson, S. (1986). *Families and Mental Handicap*. Master's dissertation, Institute of Family Therapy, London.

Todd, S., & Shearn, J. (1996). Struggles with time: The careers of parents with adult sons and daughters with learning disabilities. *Disability and Society, 1* (3): 379–401.

Todd, S., & Shearn, J. (1997). Family dilemmas and secrets. *Disability and Society, 12*: 341–366.

Tomm, K. (1984a). One perspective on the Milan approach: Part 1. Overview of development, theory and practice. *Journal of Marital and Family Therapy, 10* (2): 113–125.

Tomm, K. (1984b). One perspective on the Milan approach: Part 2. Description of session format, interviewing style and interventions. *Journal of Marital and Family Therapy, 10* (3): 253–271.

Tomm, K. (1988). Interventive interviewing Part III: Intending to ask lineal, circular, strategic, or reflexive questions. *Family Process, 27*: 1–15.

REFERENCES

Tomm, K. (1989). Externalising the problem and internalising personal agency. *Journal of Strategic and Systemic Therapies, 8*: 54–59.

Tomm, K. (1998). A question of perspective. *Journal of Marital and Family Therapy, 24* (4): 409–413.

Turnbull, A. P., Summers, J. A., & Brotherson, M. J. (1986). Family life cycle: Theoretical and empirical implications and future directions for families with mentally retarded members. In: J. Gallagher & P. Vietze (Eds.), *Families of Handicapped Persons* (pp. 58–90). Baltimore, MD: Baltimore Books.

Turner, A. L. (1980). Therapy with families of a mentally retarded child. *Journal of Marital and Family Therapy, 6*: 167–170.

Vetere, A. (1993). Using family therapy in services for people with learning disabilities. In: J. Carpenter & A. Treacher (Eds.), *Using Family Therapy in the Nineties* (pp. 111–130). Oxford: Blackwell.

Vetere, A. (1996). Soapbox: The neglect of family systems ideas in services for children and young people with learning difficulties. *Clinical Child Psychology and Psychiatry, 1*: 485–488.

Vetere, A., & Dallos, R. (2003). *Working Systemically with Families: Formulation, Intervention and Evaluation*. London: Karnac.

von Glaserfeld, E. (1987). *The Construction of Knowledge: Contributions to Conceptual Semantics*. Seaside, CA: Intersystems Publications.

Vygotsky, L. S. (1978). *Mind in Society: The Development of Higher Psychological Processes*. Cambridge, MA: Harvard University Press.

Waitman, A., & Conboy-Hill, S. (1992). *Psychotherapy and Mental Handicap*. London: Sage.

Watzlawick, P., Beavin, J., & Jackson, D. (1967). *Pragmatics of Human Communication: A Study of Interactional Patterns, Pathologies and Paradoxes*. New York: Norton.

White, M. (1984). Pseudo-encopresis: From avalanche to victory, from vicious to virtuous cycles. *Family Systems Medicine, 2* (2): 150–160.

White, M. (1989). The externalizing of the problem and the re-authoring of lives and relationships. In: M. White (Ed.), *Selected Papers* (pp. 5–28). Adelaide: Dulwich Centre Publications.

White, M. (1991). Deconstruction and therapy. *Dulwich Centre Newsletter, 3*: 21–40.

White, M. (1995). *Re-Authoring Lives: Interviews and Essays*. Adelaide: Dulwich Centre Publications.

White, M. (1997). *Narratives of Therapists' Lives*. Adelaide: Dulwich Centre Publications.

White, M. (1999). Reflecting-team work as definitional ceremony revisited. *Gecko: A Journal of Deconstruction and Narrative Ideas in Therapeutic Practice, 2*: 55–82.

White, M. (2000). *Reflections on Narrative Practice: Essays and Interviews*. Adelaide: Dulwich Centre Publications.

White, M., & Epston, D. (1990). *Narrative Means to Therapeutic Ends*. New York: Norton.

Whitney, I., Smith, P. K., & Thompson, D. (1994). Bullying and children with special educational needs. In P. K. Smith & S. Sharp (Eds.), *School Bullying* (pp. 213–40). London: Routledge.

Wikler, L., Waslow, M., & Hatfield, E. (1981). Chronic sorrow revisited: Parent versus professional depiction of the adjustment of parents of mentally retarded children. *American Journal of Orthopsychiatry, 51* (1): 63–70.

Wilcox, E., & Whittington, A. (2003). Discovering the use of narrative metaphors in work with people with learning disabilities. *Clinical Psychology, 21*: 31–35.

Wilson, J. (1998a). *Child-Focused Practice: A Collaborative Systemic Approach*. London Karnac.

Wilson, J. (1998b). Facing up to failing as a therapist: Using caricature to address therapist bias. *Human Systems, 7*: 299–311.

Wolfensberger, W. (1972). *The Principle of Normalization in Human Services*. Toronto: National Institute on Mental Retardation.

Wolfensberger, W. (1983). Social role valorization: A proposed new term for the principle of normalisation. *Mental Retardation, 21*: 234–239.

Wright, D., & Digby, A. (1996). *From Idiocy to Mental Deficiency: Historical Perspectives on People with Learning Disabilities*. London: Routledge.

Yule, W., & Carr, J. (Eds.) (1980). *Behaviour Modification for People with Mental Handicaps* (2nd edition). London: Croom Helm.

Zarkowska, E., & Clements, J. (1988). *Problem Behaviour in People with Severe Learning Disabilities*. London: Croom Helm.

INDEX

agency life-cycle stage, 147–148, 151, 162
Alcoholics Anonymous, 137
alignment, 171–174
American Association on Mental Retardation, 23
Andersen, T., 7, 13, 49, 66, 70, 85, 87–88, 125, 144–145, 173, 181, 195
Anderson, H., 85, 116, 144, 173, 179
Antaki, C., 167
anti-anorexia/bulimia league, 116–117
"approach–method–technique" model, 180
Arkless, L., 81, 183, 200
Arthur, A. R., 24, 27, 164, 168, 179
Asen, E., 28, 200
Ashcroft, J. B., 27
assessment:
　family, 89
　initial contact, 67, 68
Atkinson, L., 128
attachment:
　disorder, 128
　theory, 128
autism, 189, 196
autonomy, limits to, 129

Bank-Mikkelsen, N., 25
Barker, D., 24
Bateson, G., 49, 103, 145
Baum, S., 2–3, 10–12, 15–16, 18–20, 21–41, 64–82, 185–202
Beail, N., 27, 65
Beavers, J., 168
Beavers, R., 80
Beavers, W. R., 80, 168
Beavers Interactional Scales, 80
Beavin, J., 5, 11
behavioural approach, 27, 38
behavioural therapy, 27, 65
behaviourism, 1, 27, 130, 168

behaviour modification, 38, 168
belonging, 10, 59, 201
Bender, 27, 164, 168
Bennett, E., 66
Bennun, I., 179
Benson, M. J., 37, 90
bereavement, 76, 123, 128–129
　and loss, 76, 78
Berger, M., 75
Bertrando, P., 144
Besa, D., 117
Besley, T., 102
Bicknell, J., 33, 64
Binet, A., 22
biological systems paradigm, 8
Birmingham University, 143
Blacher, J., 29
Black, D., 36
Bloomfield, S., 173
Booth, T., 75, 114, 193, 197
Booth, W., 75, 114, 193, 197
Boscolo, L., 7, 66, 78, 144, 172
Boston, P., 121, 165
Boyd, J., 169
Boyle, B., 116
Brent, D. A., 28
Bretherton, K., 169
Bridge, S., 85
British Psychological Society, 23
　Faculty for Learning Disabilities, 19
Bromley, J., 31, 35, 37
Brotherson, M. J., 36, 177
Brown, H., 26
Brunning, H., 147
Burbach, F. R., 62
Burchardt, N., 136
Burnham, J., 9, 121, 180
Burr, V., 176
Byng-Hall, J., 135
Byrne, E. A., 29–30, 167

Cahill, J., 127
Caine, A., 27, 164, 168–169
Campbell, D., 7, 85, 103, 147, 165, 173–174
"captivated parents", 34
"captive parents", 34
Cardone, D., 11, 13–14, 17, 83–99, 195, 198–199
carer(s) (*passim*), 28
care systems, dependence upon, 58
Carey, M., 111
Carr, A., 28, 80, 84
Carr, J., 27
Carter, B., 32, 79, 168
Carter, C. O., 30
Cecchin, G., 7, 8, 66, 78, 144, 150, 172
change:
　first-order, 74–75, 201
　second-order, 75
Chapman, K., 36
Chase, J., 81, 201
choice, people's right to, 15
"chronic sorrow" of families of people with intellectual disabilities, 33, 39, 64, 78
circularity, 6, 9, 11–12
circular questions/questioning, 7, 10–11, 37, 61, 69, 72, 89, 90–92, 99, 175
"circular showing", 37
Clare, D., 101
Clegg, J., 10, 35, 79, 120–141, 165, 171, 201
Clements, J., 23, 27, 40
Cleveland, D., 31
clinical dilemmas, 170–175
Cobb, H. C., 36
co-construction, 61
co-creating meanings, 9
cognitive behavioural therapy, 18–19, 27, 65, 118, 168
Coldicott, T., 147
collaborative practice, 9, 12–13, 87
Combs, G., 4, 8–9, 66, 101–103
communication, 5–6, 9, 72, 95–98, 102, 135
　aid, electronic, 97
　attention to, 11
　book, 98
　changes in, 75
　difficulties, 11, 58, 60, 75
　disabilities, 83, 98
　facilitating:
　　drawing, showing, writing, 197
　　metaphors, stories, 199
　　photographs, video, objects, 198
　issues of, 93
　limited or inconsistent, 192
　nonverbal, 73, 84, 176
　patterns, 28, 80
　skills, lack of, 41
　verbal, 73, 84, 96
community:
　care, 25, 130, 169
　placement, 138
　team(s), 29, 42, 45, 178, 186
　disabilities, 168
　family therapy service in, 64–82
　multidisciplinary, 67, 100, 187
comprehensive process analysis, 80
Conboy-Hill, S., 168
conceptual analysis(es), 139
confidentiality, 50, 72
　issues of, 69, 74
connections in relationship, 6, 9–11
context(s):
　attending to, 6, 9–10, 28, 100, 103, 151
　concept of, 6, 9–10
　creating, 14, 88–89, 95, 97, 152
　for change, 95
　DISGRACCE, 9
　historical, 31, 35
　of individual, 9
　lifespan, 61
　multiple, 10, 103
　social, 100, 108, 115
　for systemic practice, creating, 122
contextual influences, 166, 170, 184
　on practitioners, theoretical and pragmatic, 166–170
contextualizing practice, 184
conversation(s):
　co-creating, 86
　externalizing, 104–105, 107
　"of impossibility", 16, 82
　participative, 149, 159
　　encouraging, 149–150
　reflecting-team, 7, 145
　reflective, 44, 158, 161
　therapeutic, 7–8, 106, 114, 125, 172, 199, 201
Cottrell, D., 165
Craft, A., 24
Crnic, K. A., 30
Cronen, V. E., 8, 144–145, 165–166
Crutchley, E., 85
Cummins, R., 91, 127, 131
Cunningham, C. C., 29–30, 167
curiosity, 7–9, 46, 99, 128, 173, 175
　concept of, 172
　position of, 7, 99
　respectful, 8
cybernetics:
　first-order, 5–6, 144
　second-order, 7–8, 144, 147

INDEX

Dagnan, D., 27, 91, 168
Dalal, C., 177
Dale, N., 35
Dallos, 5, 68, 165, 181
Danforth, S., 23
Daniel, G., 136
Darling, 30–31, 35
Davidson, J., 46
Davies, C. A., 167
day-service provision, 26
decisional subsystem, 173
dementia, 59, 148
Department of Health & Social Security, 15, 23, 25, 62, 85, 122, 126, 129, 154, 169, 175
de Shazer, S., 132, 178
differential power, 9–10, 14
 attention to, 9
Digby, A., 22, 27, 164, 168
discursive chaos, 140
disempowerment, 50, 61
disengagement, 120, 125, 131, 137–139
DISGRACCE, 9
Dixon, M., 36, 189
Dolan, L., 168–169
Donati, S., 164, 188
Donnellan, A. M., 27, 65
Dowling, E., 136
Dowling, M., 168–169
Downey, J., 174
Down's syndrome, 128
Draper, R., 5, 7, 85, 165, 173, 181
drawing(s), 10, 37, 73, 80, 89, 91, 106, 112, 114, 188, 197–198, 202
Drotar, D. D., 169
Dulwich Centre Publications, 117, 202

ecological systems paradigm, 7–8
Ekdawi, I., 66, 144
elaboration in the landscape:
 of action, 111
 of identity, 111
Elizur, Y., 131
Elliot, R., 8, 80
Elliott Griffith, M., 49
Ely Hospital, 25
Emerson, E., 27, 164, 168–169, 180
empowerment, 13, 15, 85
enabling participation, 191–192
enactment, 69, 167, 180
engagement, 13, 35, 37, 85, 90, 120, 125, 131–132, 137–140
epilepsy, 38, 174
Epston, D., 48, 61, 85, 92, 100–105, 112–114, 117, 138, 144–145, 171, 175–176, 201–202

ethical practices, 196
eugenics movement, 24
Eugenics Society, 22
evaluation, 62–63, 74–82, 187
 measures, 75
Evans, A., 30, 35
"expert model", 150
externalizing conversations, 104–106

family(ies), 28–31
 assessment, 89
 coping, 30
 information, recording, 89
 life cycle, 35, 10, 167
 grief and loss, 33
 issues, 177
 "out of synchrony", 33
 transitions, 32
 parental patterns, 34–35
 protection, 33
 relationship with wider systems, 35
 relationships, delineating, 89
 research:
  in intellectual disabilities, 29–30
  model, lack of, 31
 siblings, 31
 stress, 30
 structure, 5, 78, 89
  mapping, 89
 systems paradigm, 5, 7
family therapy (*passim*):
 "second-order", 85
 service, 42–65, 190, 201
  in community team, 64–82
  evaluating, 74–82
  research on, 201
 systemic, 6, 21, 29, 37, 164–165, 168, 178–180, 183, 200–201
  research studies on, 200
 vs systemic therapy, 17
 teams, lifespan, 62, 187
 vignette, 37–40
Fatimilehin, I. A., 30
Fernald, W. E., 24
Ferns, P., 26
Fidell, B., 36–37, 40, 49, 72–73, 79–80, 85–86, 88, 164, 195
Finlay, M., 167
first-order cybernetics, 5, 6, 144
Fishman, H. C., 180
Flaskas, C., 172, 180
Folkman, S., 30
Fonagy, P., 128, 183
FORSEE, 147
Foster, M., 168
fostering, 136

Foucault, M., 102, 181
Fox, H., 62, 113
Fredman, G., 1–20, 82, 86, 90, 106, 116, 136, 148, 177, 187–189, 196
Freedman, J., 4, 8–9, 66, 101–103
Freeman, J., 113–114
Friedrich, W. N., 30
Fruggeri, L., 156
Fryers, T., 22
Fuchs, K., 197
functional analysis, 27
Furlong, M., 58

Gaddis, S., 198
Gallagher, E., 164
Gangadharan, S., 169
Gardner, A., 27
Gates, R., 101
Gath, A., 31
gender roles, traditional, 125
genogram(s), 89–90, 95
Gentle, S. J., 101
George, E., 49
Gergen, K., 8, 144–145
Ghaziuddin, M., 127
Gibbons, S., 66
giving voice to people, 6, 191
Gleeson, B., 130
Glynn, B., 164
Goldberg, D., 33–37, 60, 64, 79, 85, 135, 168, 171–172, 195
Goldner, V., 129
Goolishian, H., 85, 116, 144, 173, 179
Gorell Barnes, G., 136
Grant, H., 29–30, 101
Greenberg, M. T., 30
Greenley, J. R., 30
grief, 32–34, 40, 64, 112, 167
Griffith, J. L., 8, 49
group home(s), 9, 17, 134, 188
  systemic work in, 142–163
  vignettes, 150–161
Gumley, D., 31
Gunn, W., 36
Guy, G., 46

Hailstone, E., 44
Haldipur, C. V., 127
Haley, J., 20
Halliday, S., 4, 10–15, 17, 42–63, 177, 186, 191, 200
Hampson, R. B., 80, 168
Hanley-Maxwell, C., 130
Hannah, C., 143
Hastings, R. P., 170
Hatfield, E., 33, 64, 78

Hatton, C., 27, 164, 168–169
head injury, 59
Hendy, N., 131
Hennicke, K., 23, 35–36
hermeneutics, 129
Heslop, P., 126
Hilton, A., 11, 13–14, 17, 83–99, 195, 198–199
Hoffman, L., 5, 7, 66, 84–85, 87, 144–145
Holborn, S., 130
Holmes, J., 81, 201
Hoper, J. H., 117
Houghton, B., 58
Howard, A., 130
Howe, R., 144
Hubert, J., 130
Huffington, C., 7, 147, 165, 173
Hughes, G., 66
Hulgus, Y. F., 168
Huxley, A., 142

Imber-Black, E., 35, 133
including all voices, 9, 14
inclusion, 4, 13, 26, 42–43, 85, 184, 191–192
  of client, 175–177
informed consent, issues of, 58
Ingram, J., 44, 45
intellectual disabilities (*passim*):
  definition, 2–4, 22–25
  hospitalization and segregation of people with, 24
  medicalization of, 4
intellectual disability services, 120–124, 129, 132, 133, 137, 149
intelligence quotient (IQ), 22–23
interpretative phenomenological analysis, 165
intolerance, 141
Irish Wheelchair Association, 116
issues of power and expertise, 181
Iveson, C., 49, 192–193

Jackson, D., 5, 11
Jackson, M., 25
Janssen, C., 128
Jarman, M., 165
Jay, D., 20, 25
Jay Report (1979), 25
Jenkins, R., 167
Johnson, B., 169
Jones, E., 28, 200

Kaplan, L., 173
Kars, H., 129
Kazak, A. E., 30
Kensington Consultation Centre, 28

INDEX

Kew, S., 30
Kieman, P., 167
King, S., 10, 79, 120–141, 171, 201
Kingston, P., 88
Kinsella, K., 147
Krauss, M. W., 30

Lancioni, G. E., 180
Lane, G., 8, 66, 78, 144, 150, 172
Lang, P., 8, 99, 190, 199
language:
  -based therapeutic approaches, use of, 114
  simplifying, repeating, rephrasing, 195
Lansdall-Welfare, R., 128–130
Larner, G., 117–118
La Vigna, G. W., 27, 65
Lawrence, H., 92
Lax, W., 13, 46–47
Lazarus, R. S., 30
lead practitioner, 13, 44, 46–47, 50, 57, 66–67, 70–71, 75, 86, 88, 91, 94, 96, 175, 180
  role of, 69
Learning Disability Advisory Group, 26
Leeds Family Psychology and Therapy Service (Leeds FPTS), 42–63
  nine guiding principles of, 45
  vignette, 50–55
life:
  cycle:
    family, 10, 167
    transition from childhood to adulthood, 39, 78
  planning, 154
lifespan:
  context, 61
  family therapy team(s), 43, 46, 47, 61, 62, 187
  service, development of, 43–45
lifestyles, restricted, 58
Lindsay, W., 91
linguistic systems paradigm, 8
Lobovits, D., 113, 114
Lowe, E., 46
Lussardi, D. J., 46
Lynggaard, H., 10, 13, 15–20, 36–37, 92, 100–119, 164, 176, 185–202
Lyons, E., 167

Madsen, W. C., 131–132
Makaton symbols, 98
Martin, D., 37, 90
Martin, R. S., 30
Mason, B., 123, 174
material resources, role of, 18

Matthews, B., 101
Matthews, S., 36, 189
Mattison, V., 197
Maturana, H., 179
McAdam, E., 8, 99, 190, 199
McCarthy, J., 169
McCarthy, M., 26
McCollum, E., 72
McConachie, H., 168
McGoldrick, M., 32, 79, 168
McGrath, M., 30
McIntosh, P., 24, 170
McLachlan, D., 58
McNamee, S., 8, 144
Meakes, E., 117
meaning(s):
  co-creating, 9, 102
  patterns of, 7
memory problems, 58, 191
Mental Deficiency Act (1913), 22
Mental Health Foundation, 26
mental health needs assessment, 42
metaphor(s), 4–8, 61, 89, 92–95, 133, 176, 199
  narrative, 8, 103
  use of, 92, 199
  vignette, 92–95
Midence, K., 35
Milan method, 44
Milan systemic therapy, 44, 66, 78, 85, 103, 143, 165
Miller, N., 31
Minuchin, S., 66, 103, 180
"miracle question", 178
Mitchell, W., 30, 36, 169
Mittler, P., 169
modernism, 5
Moon, S. M., 75, 80, 201
Morgan, A., 49, 101, 109, 111–114, 116
multidisciplinary setting, referrals in, 189
multidisciplinary team(s) (MDT), 145–146, 148–151, 156
multiple narratives, 139
multiple perspectives, 7–9, 13, 46, 61, 92, 122, 147, 188
multiple realities, 120, 125, 129, 136, 140
Murray, K., 92

Nadirshaw, Z., 30
narrative(s):
  approach(es), 16, 66, 104, 114–115, 119
  metaphor, 8, 103
  multiple, 139
  therapy, 92, 100–119, 176
National Health Service (NHS), 45, 83, 121–122, 145

negotiation, process of, 74
Neilson, C., 91
neutrality, concept of, 172
Newham family therapy service in community team, 64–82
"news of difference", 92, 145, 162
Nielsen, S., 173
Nirje, B., 25
"non-expert" model, 85, 89, 145, 147, 155, 180
normalization, 4, 6, 15, 25–27, 126, 130, 169, 180
  ideology of, 25
"not-knowing position", 85, 145
Nottinghamshire Healthcare NHS Trust, 121

O'Brien, J., 25, 169
Oliver, P. C., 183, 200
one-way mirror/screen, 18, 44, 46, 48, 66–67, 82, 121, 145, 187
O'Reilly, M. F., 180
organizational life cycle, concept of, 173
organizational settings, 147
Osbeck, L., 127
Osborn, M., 165
outcome tools, 75
out-of-synchrony life-cycle events, 32–33, 64
outsider-witness groups, 146
Owens, R. J., 27
Oxford Family Institute, 143

paradigm:
  biological systems, 8
  ecological systems, 7, 8
  family systems, 5, 7
  linguistic systems, 8
"participant observer", 144, 145
participative conversations, 149, 159
Partridge, K., 66
Pascall, G., 131
paternalism, 50, 60
Paterson, S., 85
patterns of meaning, 7
Pearce, B. W., 165–166
Pearce, P., 164, 188
Pearson, M., 121
peer supervision, 189
Penn, P., 7, 66
People First, 171
Percy, I., 110
"perfect child", grief for loss of, 33, 64, 167
Perlesz, A., 58, 85, 172
"perpetual parenthood", 32, 34
  anxiety about, 64

Perry, L., 101
person-centred planning (PCP), 130–131, 154–156
person-centred practice, 13, 85
perspectives, multiple, 7–9, 13, 46, 61, 92, 122, 147, 188
phenomenological analysis, interpretative, 165
Pickering, M. R., 117
Pogoloff, S., 130
positivism, 5
post-Milan therapy, 66, 78, 165
post-reflection conversation, 48–49
Pote, H., 10, 16, 164–184, 189, 191, 196, 200–201
Potts, M., 130
power and expertise, issues of, 181
  vignette, 181–183
Prata, G., 172
problem-determined system(s), 173–175, 184
  definition, 175
  identifying, 184
  mapping, vignette, 174–175
problem-saturated story(ies)/views of self, 47, 58–59, 101, 103, 105, 108–109, 115, 149
process research, 165
professional training, therapists', 166, 168, 184
protection:
  issue of, 10, 32–34, 59–60, 125, 136, 167
  triangles of, 171, 173
psychodynamic therapy, 19, 38, 65, 168
psychotherapeutic models of therapy, 27

Quarry, A., 62
questions/questioning, circular, 7, 10, 11, 72, 89, 90, 92, 99, 175

Race, D., 22, 23, 25, 29
randomized controlled trials, 183
Rapley, M., 167
Ratner, H., 49
Raval, H., 68, 69
Ray, W., 8, 66, 78, 144, 150, 172
Real, T., 46
Reder, P., 90, 148, 177
reflecting conversation(s), 14, 44, 152–153, 157–158, 161, 175
reflecting team(s) (*passim*):
  conversations, 7, 47, 145
  method, 44, 57, 88
  role of, 69–70
reflective processes, 49, 178
  vignette, 178–179

reflexivity, 88, 172, 173
Reid, D. H., 169
Reinders, H. S., 129
"relational knowing", 195
relationship map, 90, 96, 97
relativism, 8
Remington, B., 170
reparative script, 135
research:
   modern and postmodern views of, 117
   need for, 183–184
   primary and secondary, 117
   process, systemic therapy, 165
   projects, service-orientated, 44
   randomized control, 116
   role of, 139
   on systemic approaches, 199–202
residential care, 138
residential homes, 28, 29
resistance, 132
responsibility, 10, 36, 163
Rhodes, J., 62
Rhodes, P., 164, 168, 177
Rikberg Smyly, S., 10, 12, 14–15, 17, 27, 29, 142–163, 173, 188, 199
risk, 10, 59, 140
   and independent living, 171
Risley, T. R., 169
Robbins, L., 4, 10–12, 14–15, 17, 42–63, 177, 186, 191, 200
Roccoforte, J. A., 30
Rose, N., 128
Roth, A., 105, 112, 183
Roy-Chowdhury, S., 36, 73, 78
Ruddick, L., 91
Russell, S., 111
Ryan, J., 3, 127

Sabat, S. R., 191
Saetersdal, B., 131
Salmon, A., 36–37, 164
"scaffolding", 196, 197
scapegoating, 60, 73, 78
Schaefer, C., 30
Schindler-Zimmerman, T., 37, 90
Schuengel, C., 128
Schuman, M., 117
Scior, K., 10, 13, 15, 17–18, 36–37, 92, 100–119, 164, 176, 188
second-order cybernetics, 7, 8, 144, 147
second-order practice, 85
Seikkula, S., 200
self-advocacy, 26
self-reflexivity, 8, 165, 172, 175, 177, 184, 196
self-report measures, 80

Seligman, M., 30, 31, 35
Seltzer, M. M., 29, 30
Selvini Palazzoli, M. S., 172
separation, 10, 59, 128, 136
service development, recommendations for, 62
Shapiro, D., 165
Sheard, C., 127–128
Shearn, J., 34, 64, 78, 130
Sheppard, N., 36
Shotter, J., 195
Shulman, S., 31, 36
siblings, 31
Simon, T., 22
Simons, K., 26, 126
Sinason, V., 27, 34, 61, 65, 130, 164, 168–169
Skelly, A., 129
Sklavounos, D., 188
Sloper, P., 30, 36, 169
Smith, D., 88
Smith, H., 26
Smith, J., 165
Smith, P. K., 127
Snyder, W., 72
social constructionism, 8, 35, 83–85, 102, 143–147, 181, 188
social inclusion, 4, 26
social role valorization, 25
Sonuga-Barke, J. S., 170
Speedy, J., 201–202
Sprague, S., 117
Sprenkle, D. H., 75, 80, 201
Stack, L. S., 127
staff team, beliefs, attitudes, expectations of, 148–149
Stenfert Kroese, B., 27, 65, 168
St James-O'Connor, T., 117
Stolk, J., 128, 129
story(ies):
   alternative, 15, 48, 110, 112, 145, 149
   new, 14, 105, 110–111, 144–147, 163
   consolidating and extending, 111–113
   staff, 154
Stratton, P., 165
Street, E., 174
structuralism, 5
structural therapy, 66, 180
Sturm, L. A., 169
Sugden, C., 197
suicide, 125
Summers, J. A., 36, 177
supervision, 67, 71
   peer, 189
   systemic, 82, 186
supported living, 26, 28

symbol(s), 37, 73, 80, 89, 91
    Makaton, 98
systemic approach(es) (*passim*):
    definition, 4–5
    effectiveness of, 199–202
    postmodern, 8
systemic family therapy, 6, 21, 29, 37,
    164–168, 178–180, 183, 200–201
systemic practice (*passim*):
    first phase, 5
systemic principles, 5, 8–9, 103
systemic supervision, 82, 186
systemic therapeutic service, clinic-based,
    84
systemic therapy (*passim*):
    vs family therapy, 17
    Milan, 44, 66, 78, 85, 103, 143, 165
    practitioner's position and dilemmas,
        164–184
    process research, 165
    service, setting up, 65–75
    vignette, 95–98
systems paradigm:
    biological, 8
    ecological, 7, 8
    family, 5, 7
    linguistic, 8

Tench, C., 62
therapeutic conversations, 7–8, 106, 114,
    125, 172, 199, 201
therapeutic letter(s), 113, 138
Thomas, B., 129
Thomas, F., 3
Thompson, D., 127
Thompson, H., 127
Thompson, P., 136
Thomson, S., 36
time, concept of, 197
Todd, S., 34, 64, 78, 130
Tomm, K., 7, 48, 90, 103
transition(s) (*passim*):
    from childhood to adulthood, 39, 78,
        135–136, 167
    experiences, vignettes, 133–140
    interventions, 120
    literature review, 126–132

planning, 126
policy and research, 126–128
life-cycle, 21, 32–36, 39–40, 78, 127
Turnbull, A. P., 36, 177
Turner, A. L., 36

United Kingdom Council for
    Psychotherapy (UKCP), 165

Vetere, A., 31, 33, 35–36, 64, 68, 167–168
Vietze, P., 130
visual aid(s), 37, 80
voices, including all, 14–15
von Foerster, H., 144
von Glaserfeld, E., 102
Vygotsky, L. S., 196

Waitman, A., 168
Walden, S., 11, 18–19, 36, 64–82, 186, 198,
    201
Waslow, M., 33, 64, 78
Watzlawick, P., 5, 11
Webster, A., 66
White, M., 45, 48–49, 61, 85, 92, 100–104,
    109, 113, 116–117, 122, 138, 144–146,
    171–172, 175–176, 201
White Papers:
    *Better Services for the Mentally
        Handicapped* (1971), 23, 25
    Fulfilling the Promises (Wales, 2001), 26
    The Same as You? (Scotland, 2000), 26
    Valuing People (England, 2001, 2002), 4,
        26, 62, 85, 122, 126, 129, 154, 171,
        175, 187
Whitney, I., 127, 130
Whitney-Thomas, J., 130
Whittington, A., 101
Wikler, L., 33, 64, 78
Wilcox, E., 101
Wilson, J., 132–133, 176, 191
Wolfensberger, W., 4, 25, 169
Wright, D., 22, 27, 164, 168

Young, J., 58, 85
Yule, W., 27

Zarkowska, E., 27

Nikki Swan